D1378735

Family and Individual Development

Contributions to Human Development

Vol. 14

Series Editor
J.A. Meacham, Buffalo, N.Y.

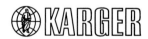

Basel · München · Paris · London · NewYork · New Delhi · Singapore · Tokyo · Sydney

Family and Individual Development

Volume Editor
J.A. Meacham, Buffalo, N.Y.

6 figures and 1 table, 1985

WITHDRAWN

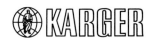

Basel · München · Paris · London · NewYork · New Delhi · Singapore · Tokyo · Sydney

Contributions to Human Development

National Library of Medicine, Cataloging in Publication
Family and individual development /
volume editor, J.A. Meacham. -- Basel; New York: Karger, 1985. --
(Contributions to human development; vol. 14)
Includes bibliographies and indexes.
1. Family   2. Human Development   I. Meacham, J.A.   II. Series
W1 CO778S v. 14 [BF 713 F198]
ISBN 3-8055-4037-X

© Copyright 1985 by S. Karger AG, P.O. Box, CH-4009 Basel (Switzerland)
Printed in Switzerland by Thür AG Offsetdruck, Pratteln
ISBN 3-8055-4037-X

Contents

Preface

Family and individual development are considered in the present volume within the context of cultural change and within the framework of life-span developmental psychology. Among the topics woven together in the various chapters are parenting behaviors, development of personality and sex roles, relations between grandparents, children, and grandchildren, psychological development in adulthood and late adulthood, cultural change, and service delivery. The authors' conclusions are based in research with groups as diverse as the Druse of the Middle East, Irish, Italian, and Polish immigrants to the United States, and rural elderly in West Virginia. A variety of conceptual frameworks are represented, including Wernerian, psychodynamic, Eriksonian, etc. Despite this diversity, the authors agree on the need to investigate human development not within isolated individuals, but as development occurs within a life-span developmental framework including the individual's life course, the lives of family members from other generations, and the changing cultural and historical context. This volume will be of interest to psychologists, sociologists, and anthropologists, as well as to students of family theory and practice.

What is life-span developmental psychology? A common view, but one that is incomplete, is that life-span developmental psychology is merely the study of psychological development over the life span, from birth to death, through infancy, childhood, adolescence, adulthood, and aging. This view is reflected in the addition to many standard texts on child and adolescent development of a final chapter on adulthood, supposedly transforming these texts from child development texts into life-span development texts. There is often much that is good within these revised texts, such as rejection of parallels between physical growth and decline and psychological development, and recognition of the fact that psychological development may progress in many directions along various dimensions throughout adulthood. But life-span developmental psychology is much more than this.

Life-span developmental psychology is the study of psychological development within multiple contexts, including the life course itself, the social context, and the encompassing cultural and historical context. These multiple contexts are not merely the backdrop against which the drama of individual development unfolds; rather, they represent dynamic processes with a developmental history of their own. Thus, from a life-span developmental perspective, stages of life such as childhood or adulthood cannot be studied in isolation from each other, first one and then the next, as the chapters in a text are sequenced. Instead, each stage of life must be understood in the context of developmental changes within all the others. For example, the activities of childhood and adolescence reflect in large part anticipation of and preparation for the tasks of work and family in adulthood, and the construction of a meaningful existence in adulthood and old age reflects in part a reworking of the goals and ideals of youth (Helen Kivnick refers to these processes in her chapter as previewing and renewing). From a life-span developmental perspective, the social context of the family is not merely the backdrop for child development. Instead, the development of each member of the family and of each generation of the family must be understood in relation to developmental changes within all the others. Not only do parents structure the development of their children, but – as David Gutmann and Helen Kivnick argue in their chapters in this volume – the children structure the further development of the parents. From a life-span developmental perspective, the cultural and historical context is not merely a geographical variable, to be considered in a separate chapter on cross-cultural differences. Instead, this context is a temporal variable, developing in its own right at the same time that families and individual persons are developing within it.

The subject matter of life-span developmental psychology is not an isolated individual, developing along an idealized progression within static family and cultural contexts [*Riegel and Meacham*, 1976]. Instead, all the family members – the children, the parents, the grandparents – continue to develop simultaneously, in relation to and in reaction to each other, and the cultural context similarly continues to change around the developing individuals and families, and in reaction to the development of individuals and families. It becomes difficult to specify the locus of development as solely within the individual. In some cases the appearance of individual development may reflect no changes at all within the individual, but rather multiple changes in the relationship between the individual and the changing family and cultural context. For example, are the apparent developmental changes of adulthood and old age best understood as changes within individuals who are aging within a relatively static family and cultural context, or as lack of change within individuals who live in a context of rapid social and cultural change? The subject matter of life-span developmental psychology is not an isolated, developing individual, but the changing relations between developing individuals, the changing social context of the family, and the developing cultural and historical context [*Meacham,* 1984]. Individuals change, families change, and the cultural context changes, each in relation to and in reaction to the others.

All of these themes are expressed and illustrated within the present volume, which focuses on the relations between developing individuals and developing families within changing cultural contexts. Judith and Frank Hooper conclude in the first chapter that the developing family unit plays a central role in linking patterns of development within individuals with changes at the societal level. (This conclusion is illustrated in the following chapter by David Gutmann.) They suggest that certain conceptual and methodological difficulties in bringing together primarily sociological family theories with primarily psychological theories of individual development may be resolved by adopting the general framework of Heinz Werner's developmental theory. Family development theories will need to take into consideration such psychological variables as belief systems, family history and myth, and the meaning of roles and role-taking, and both family and individual development theories will need to accommodate the fact that the nuclear family, as a result of larger societal changes, may be becoming a thing of the past.

David Gutmann argues that the state of parenthood within the context of the family, with children's demands for meeting their physical and emotional needs, drives the individual developmental changes of adulthood, including the sharpening of sex roles during parenthood and the release of latent potentials during the postparental years. Further, these developments of the postparental years are essential to maintenance of the society and of the species, so that postparental parents are better viewed as emeritus parents than as ex-parents. The role for women changes from one of direct, primary care of infants and children to an executive or administrative role, managing the extended family and its parental couples, insuring the continuity of the family's trust, traditions, and reliable parenting. The role for older men becomes less one of maintaining the physical security of the family, and more one of maintaining the ritual and spiritual resources of the family and of the broader community and society. In sum, Gutmann argues, it is changes such as these, and not adaptation to loss, that constitute the nature of individual development in later life and of species preservation. The cultural context, rather than being merely a backdrop for family and individual development, is maintained by these developments.

Gutmann's focus on relations between children and parents is extended in the remaining chapters, all of which consider intergenerational relations in varying cultural contexts. These chapters were initially prepared for a symposium organized by Jeanne Thomas for the annual meeting of the Gerontological Society of America. Bertram Cohler considers personality and family development in the context of rapid social change, in particular, immigration from Europe to the United States. Considerable variation is found in intergenerational relations as a function of national origin and length of time in the United States. For example, for Irish and Italian ethnic groups, the position of older parents within the family has shown dramatic reversals – for the Irish, the power of older parents has been reduced; for the Italians, the power has been enhanced. For Italian-Americans, there are stronger expectations than for other ethnic groups for older parents to continue to be actively engaged in caring for others. In the following chapter, Dean Rodeheaver points to the long-term impact of parent-child relationships even as the parents progress into later adulthood, by locating these relationships in the context of use of social support networks in the changing culture of a rural area.

The concluding chapters are concerned with grandparenthood, as a reaction to the changing circumstances of younger generations, and as an impetus for further developmental change. Jeanne Thomas and Nancy Datan report the results of interviews with grandparents regarding their perceptions of relationships with their grandchildren, and how these relationships and the roles for grandparents change as a function of the grandchildren's development. In parallel with Gutmann's argument that adult development is structured by the needs of children, Helen Kivnick argues in the concluding chapter that development in later adulthood is structured by grandparents' continuing involvement in the family cycle – in the middle adulthood of their own children, and in the childhood and adolescence of their grandchildren. To the extent that grandparents are able to promote psychosocial development in their children and grandchildren, they are also effective in promoting their own development, especially in terms of the

Eriksonian crises of generativity and intimacy. The themes of this volume are nicely summarized in Kivnick's concluding sentence, which calls for understanding the process of living life as an individual, in a family, in a society, and in history.

References

Meacham, J.A.: The individual as consumer and producer of historical change; in McCluskey, Reese, Life-span developmental psychology: historical and generational effects (Academic Press, New York 1984).

Riegel, K.F.; Meacham, J.A.: The developing individual in a changing world (Mouton, The Hague 1976).

Contr. hum. Dev., vol. 14, pp. 1–30 (Karger, Basel 1985)

Family and Individual Developmental Theories: Conceptual Analysis and Speculations

Judith O. Hooper, Frank H. Hooper

University of Wisconsin-Madison, Madison, Wisc., USA

It may be contended that although sociologically and psychologically oriented theories of development are inextricably related, they seem to be doomed to passively separate existences. For the case of family and individual development at least, this appears to be true in many university settings. Thus, family research and theory is usually found in administrative units separate from other observers of human development across the life span, especially from those who espouse an experimental psychological orientation (see *Hill* [1979] and *Wohlwill* [1973, pp. 376–380] for a provocative discussion of the high degree of academic specialization and lack of interdisciplinary cooperation in most United States universities). Yet the fact remains that the great majority of individuals enter the world, develop to maturity, and pass away in a family setting. Surely each discipline has a great deal of information to convey to the other.

Hill and Mattessich [1979] have attempted to foster interdisciplinary collaboration between family developmental theorists and the group of scholars primarily concerned with individual development, including social gerontologists. They are certainly to be commended for this attempt to 'blend' one version of family theory with an enormous range of additional conceptual speculation and associated empirical research findings. We believe this integrative endeavor to be long overdue.

However, our current appreciation for the inherent complexities in each theoretical domain (family theory and models which are primarily of a sociological nature versus theories of individual human development across the life span) and for the considerable methodological difficulties faced by each suggests certain important caveats [e.g., *Bengtson,* 1977;

Featherman, 1983]. The purpose of the present chapter is to build upon the initial *Hill and Mattessich* suggestions, and to explicate some of the problems and shortcomings as well as the strong points in expanding family developmental theory to encompass other developmental models and research. We believe that the current version of family development theory may suffer from certain problems of internal and external validity [*Cook and Campbell,* 1979; *Campbell and Stanley,* 1963] which arise from the implicit attempt to blend aspects of the original family model with organismic individual developmental theory. Problems of external validity primarily concern the generalizability [cf. *Campbell and Stanley,* 1963, p. 5] of the family development model as it applies to modern conditions. Generalizability is to be viewed as involving both across-situation consistency and across-sample similarity vis-à-vis the possible populations of families in a given sociocultural milieu. In brief, we are concerned that the family development model, as it is presently formulated, may have explanatory power for fewer and fewer families [e.g., *Edelman,* 1981; *Feldman and Feldman,* 1975; *Segalen,* 1974; *Spanier* et al., 1975; *Trost,* 1973].

Organismic Theory and Family Developmental Theory

The main question was succinctly stated by *Hill and Mattessich* as follows:

> The major point of confrontation between conceptualizers of family development and developmental psychology comes from examining the assumptions of different models about the phenomenon of development. ... Is there any isomorphism either between 'development' over the life span of humans as biosocial organisms and the 'development' of families as they form and change in function and structure over their life history or between these two phenomena and 'development' in larger aggregations of communities and whole societies over time? [*Hill and Mattissich,* 1979, p. 172].

Hill and Mattessich [1979, pp. 178–179] offer a conceptual analysis of the most popular individual developmental theories [adapted from *Looft,* 1973, and *Lerner,* 1978] and add to this array the family development approach.

In 7 of the 10 model issues discussed, the family development approach and general organismic theory (as exemplified by the work of Werner, Piaget, Kohlberg, and Erikson) had identical or very similar entries. The exceptions included closed versus open models, the nature of individual or individual-family differences, and the directionality of development. It may thus be assumed that the family development approach is closer to the organismic approach than to the so-called 'mechanistic' models [*Peterson* et al., 1979]. Thus, *Hill and Mattessich* [1979, p. 172] commented, '... These views of the primacy of individuals as initiators rather than solely reactors are more compatible with developmental theorists who use the organismic model ... than the social learning theory psychologists who espouse the mechanistic model ...'.

Throughout this discussion, we are assuming that all models and derivative theories may be evaluated in terms of six basic criteria: (a) the degree of logical internal consistency; (b) the degree of coverage or scope included by the model; (c) the degree of parsimony; (d) the external validity or degree of correspondence with empirical data of the model; (e) the potential implications for the human condition or the implied ethics of the models in question, and (f) the functional utility or heuristic value of the model as a general source for *future* research and theorizing. The first four of these criteria were initially presented in the 1890s by Heinrich Hertz in his *Principles of Mechanics* [cf. *Janik and Toulmin,* 1973, pp. 141–142]. We might also add the special rules of falsifiability, relevance, and independence or noncircularity [cf. *Brainerd,* 1981, p. 66]. An inordinate emphasis on one criterion (internal consistency excepted) usually results in a diminishing of the other criteria, e.g., parsimony versus scope. Indeed, some writers [e.g. *Lachman,* 1960; *Looft,* 1973; *Overton and Reese,* 1973; *Reese and Overton,* 1970] have argued that since the fundamental truth criteria differ, the only valid distinction among contrasting metamodels or world views concerns the last-named heuristic function. Although counter-arguments to this position [originally proposed by *Pepper,* 1942] have been offered [e.g., *Beilin,* 1983; *Merlino,* 1975; *Overton,* 1983; *Page and Smither*], it is evident that *Hill and Mattessich* freely borrow from a number of metamodels of individual development in their suggestions for 'reconstructing' family developmental theory.

Thoughts concerning the potential complementarity of family models and organismic models in general and Piaget's theory in particular are certainly not new. As long ago as 1938, *Waller,* in discussing the essential social origins of reflective consciousness, wrote:

It is to be regretted that Piaget did not also study his subjects' home environment. It seems more than likely that a great deal of what Piaget was forced to consider egocentric conversation would have appeared in a different light if the child could have been observed against the background of family appreciation. The egocentricity of the child may be a function of his life in the family, where he does not need to take the role of the other because the others are only too ready to make all the adjustments to him. The egocentricity of the child does not, in the family environment, amount to an indifference to, or ignorance of, the attitudes of others toward him. When children trained in the ordinary family environment go to school, it is only to be expected that they would behave in the manner which Piaget describes.

Piaget's studies seem to substantiate Mead's central point. Mind as we know it is a social product. Our minds are greatly influenced by the culture which is mediated to us in the communicative process. Logic, and submission to logic and reality, are results of taking the role of the other, and of a laboriously established participation in a common life. On this point the interpretations of Piaget, Mead, Dewey, Cooley, Freud, Ferenczi, Durkheim, MacIver, and many others seem to converge [p. 52].

Piaget recognized the need to coordinate ontogenetic and sociological analyses [cf. *Piaget,* 1960, pp. 8–9; 1970, pp. 97–128; 1972, pp. 359–361, 368–369]. He is quoted by *Hill* [1979] as having said, 'If I had thirty years to live again, I would start looking at families. The basic task, however, is description ... not yet explanation'.

Changes in family structure with the concomitant changes in role relationships [e.g., *Kreppner* et al., 1982; *Parish and Parish,* 1983], as well as the more obvious changes from family situation to a school environment may be examined in terms of structure/function or means/ends relationships in early childhood. From the organismic perspective it is not until new functional demands are made upon the child (e.g., in the school setting) that concomitant cognitive structural changes will gradually take place. These novel structures, in turn, permit an extended range of functional adaptation. In this regard, it is interesting to note that a number of research investigations have highlighted the role of family structure variables and related social factors as likely determinants of children's cognitive functioning from the Piagetian perspective [e.g., *Hollos,* 1975; *Hollos and Cowan,* 1973; *McGillicuddy* et al., 1979; *Reid,* 1984].

Our initial concern involves the definition of a developmental event for the two approaches. Thus we can compare *Hill and Mattesich* [1979, p. 174]:

Family development refers to the process of progressive structural differentiation and transformation over the family's history, to the active acquisition and selective discarding of roles by incumbents of family positions as they seek to meet the changing functional requisites for survival and as they adapt to recurring life stresses as a family system;

with *Nagel* [1957, pp. 16–17]:

> ... the term (development) is reserved for changes which are not merely irreversible, or which yield only a greater numerical complexity; those changes must in addition eventuate in modes of organization not previously manifested in the history of the developing system, such that the system acquires an increased capacity for self-regulation, a larger measure of relative independence from environmental fluctuations ... (and further) the connotation of *development* thus involves two essential components: the notion of a system possessing a definite structure and a definite set of pre-existing capacities; and the notion of a sequential set of changes in the system, yielding relatively permanent but novel increments not only in its structure but in its modes of operation as well.

Can we surmise from these definitions that both approaches are primarily concerned with *qualitative* changes in the *form* or organization of the systems in question, in contrast to the sheer number, strength, or accuracy of the roles, the responses, or the behaviors? Assuming the answer to be affirmative, we can now examine the particular nature and, most importantly, the causal determinants of these developmental changes.

Perhaps a more parsimonious way to view these distinctions is by examining the basic forms of causation held to be operative by the various models and world views. It is commonly acknowledged that the mechanistic world view accepts two forms of causation, material and efficient. Material causes of an object or event are the substances which constitute the object in question. 'Granting historical changes in the scientific conception of substance, a present-day example of material causes would consist of the physiological, neurological, or genetic substrate that is a necessary condition for behavior. Efficient cause is the external agent, antecedent condition, or independent variable which moves the object (causes the event)' [*Overton and Reese,* 1973, p. 75]. Although they do not specifically mention them, we assume that *Hill and Mattessich* [1979, table 1, p. 179] would accept material causes. They definitely accept efficient causation of the antecedent-consequent variety.

Organicists, of course, insist upon two additional causal types, formal and final. 'Formal cause is the pattern, organization, or form of an object. Thus, the specification of psychological structures, for example, constitutes a formal cause' [*Overton and Reese,* 1973, p. 75]. Insofar as they accept structural/functional analysis, *Hill and Mattessich* appear to acknowledge the importance of formal causation. Their acceptance of final causation, in contrast, seems somewhat problematic. Final causes may involve two concepts, the specification of an end toward which the individual or system develops (as in the classic view of a closed system), and/or a superordinate, developmental factor such as Piaget's equilibration process. It is a moot question at this point whether the family system according to *Hill* is best viewed as an open or closed entity (it appears to be 'becoming' more open as subsequent versions of his theory indicate, e.g., compare *Hill and Rodgers* [1964] with *Hill and Mattessich* [1977, pp. 2, 38, and footnote 2, and 1979, pp. 179, 198]. However, the final causes are openly teleological in nature and we are not sure whether *Hill* would agree that family systems are *always* developing toward some endpoint or goal.

In all fairness to *Hill's* apparent equivocality concerning closed systems, it should be mentioned that *Piaget's* views on this issue also appeared to change. Without de-emphasizing the importance of the formal period of logical thought as an endpoint toward which cognitive development is directed, *Piaget* (and his recent interpreters) came to acknowledge a number of interesting developments during the mature adult years [e.g., *Chandler,* 1975; *Edelstein and Noam,* 1982; *Kramer,* 1983; *Labouvie-Vief,* 1980, 1982; *Piaget,* 1972; *Riegel,* 1973]. Nonetheless, organicists such as *Piaget* and *Werner* are adamant in insisting that the complete picture of development must include all four causal determinants as outlined above [*Overton and Reese,* 1981].

One of the major implications of this insistence by the organicists is the recognition (in direct opposition to the mechanists, of course) that teleological laws are viewed as basic and therefore *not* ultimately reducible to efficient causal laws. They in fact *subsume* efficient and material causal determinants [*Overton and Reese,* 1973, p. 83]. This results in an emphasis upon reciprocal rather than unidirectional causality, and organized complexity rather than linear and additive causality. One specific example of this concerns the transition sequence processes across the major Piagetian stages or periods of development. The principle of *emergent* development '... implies that later stage-related behavioral manifestations cannot be exhaustively predicted or causally linked from information specific to earlier modes of responding although the converse relationship may hold' [*F. Hooper,* 1973, p. 304].

One often gets the impression of the family development model that, although the cycles or stages are said to be qualitatively discrete, the process mechanisms which govern change are quantitative, continous, additive, and linear in nature. This is shown by the emphasis upon such factors as the time since marriage, the number of children per family unit, the chronological ages of the siblings, and the age spacing or density among the siblings.

Representative stage descriptions for the family development model include:

I   beginning families (couples married less than 5 years with no children);
II   childbearing families (oldest child, birth to 2 years, 11 months);
III   families with preschool children (oldest child, 3–5 years, 11 months);
IV   families with school-age children (oldest child, 6–12 years,
       11 months);
V   families with teenagers (oldest child, 13–20 years, 11 months);
VI   families as launching centers (first child gone to last child leaving
       home);
VII   families in the middle years (empty nest to retirement), and
VIII aging families (retirement to death of first spouse) [from *Spanier* et al.,
       1975; table 2, p. 270; see also *Duvall*, 1971; table 6–5, p. 151].

One might well ask whether the changes which are represented by the family stages are cases of quantitative or qualitative discontinuity [cf. *Page and Smither*, unpubl. data, pp. 110–120; *Werner and Kaplan*, 1973]. If they are 'prototypes' of qualitative discontinuity then they should meet the general requirements of stages or levels in organismic theory.

A Special Case: Family and Individual Developmental Stages

Stages of development have apparently long held a peculiar fascination for obervers of the human condition [*Glaserfeld and Kelly*, 1982; *Kessen*, 1962]. The conceptual use of the term stage varies widely among various writers, however. Thus, when *Bijou and Baer* [1961] use stages, they designate only *descriptive* categories [cf. *Brainerd*, 1978, pp. 173–174]. Some writers use stages in a weaker general metaphorical sense as shown by the 'chimpanzee stage' or as a paraphrase for age, e.g., 'the terrible two's'. Certain learning theorists use the term as a rough age demarcation for the absence versus the presence of certain behavioral capacities, e.g., the verbal mediation theorists such as *Reese* or the *Kendlers*. *Bruner's* [1964] stages or levels of development, the enactive, the iconic, and the symbolic, also follow this pattern. As is the case with *Gagne's* [1968] hierarchial learning model, the transitions across the various stages and levels are viewed in a strictly additive fashion and complete antecedent-consequent causation is assumed to govern the task analysis sequences. In marked contrast, the organismic writers employ a much stronger usage of the stage construct, one which has a clear commitment to biological foundations (e.g., Piaget and Freud).

For most American writers, developmental process mechanisms have held less appeal while stages and developmental periods remain the best known and most controversial component of the Piagetian system. Conceptual analyses of the Genevan version of developmental stages include essays by *Beilin* [1971], *Bickhard* [1978], *Brainerd* [1978, 1979, 1981], *Feldman and Toulmin* [1976], *Flavell* [1971, 1981, 1982], *F. Hooper* [1973], *Pinard and Laurendeau* [1969], *Toulmin* [1971], and *Wohlwill* [1973]. These accounts have highlighted the theoretical emphases and associated empirical issues associated with stages as descriptive, metaphorical, and (potentially) explanatory constructs. *Piaget* [1960, 1970a, b] identifies four major criteria for cognitive stages: hierarchization, consolidation, integration and structuring, and equilibration. Hierarchization refers to the well-known postulate of stage invariance or transitivity of progression throughout the developmental sequence. Later stages or levels can never precede the earlier acquisitions; i.e., in the sequence of stages A–B–C–D, all individuals demonstrate C capabilities after stage B and prior to stage D. Integration (per se) is a closely related concept which specifies that subsequent stages or levels transform earlier stage behavior into new structural entities. Prior stages are not simply replaced (in an additive or substitutive fashion), but rather become subordinated and subsumed within the higher-level functioning. This last property or attribute of stage progressions concerns the emergence assumptions of Piaget's theory that are shared by all organismic viewpoints [cf. *Kaplan*, 1967; *Nagel*, 1957; *Overton and Reese*, 1973, 1981; *Reese and Overton*, 1970].

Consolidation refers to the fact that each stage or period has a preparatory and stabilization phase associated with it (indeed, each intermediate stage in the Piagetian system is viewed as the culmination of all those that have come before and the starting point of all those to follow). Early stage-specific behaviors are transitory and reminiscent of the earlier modes of functioning. Typically, old means (structures) are applied to new ends or functional demands [*Werner*, 1957]. Gradually the child's new response repertory becomes generalized and more stable, which in turn sets the stage for the next developmental transition via the equilibration dynamic.

The structural and integration assumptions are unquestionably the most salient aspects of a meaningful stage designation for Piaget. All the organizational simplicity and potential explanatory parsimony follows from the *structures d'ensemble* postulate. As stated previously:

The behavioral outcomes of this assumption are numerous – for example, interrelationships between responses to different tasks involving the same operations [*Wohlwill*, 1963], operational convergence [*Beilin*, 1965], functional correspondence [*F. Hooper*,

1973], significant interitem correlations [*Braine,* 1959; *Shantz,* 1967], complete functional interdependence and organic connections [*Pinard and Laurendeau,* 1969], concurrences [*Flavell,* 1970, 1971], and interpatterning among sets of developing responses [*Wohlwill,* 1973]. All of these outcomes highlight the intra-individual and inter-individual uniformity across response domains that is to be expected of persons 'located' in a given stage of development. Moreover, contrary to *Brainerd's* conclusions, the *integration* assumption implies more than a merely additive notion that each successive stage includes the earlier stage's dominant response prototypes. Rather, later and more complex stages effectively transform and reorganize the earlier stages into new functional entities. Lower-order responses become subordinated as higher stages are achieved, and they assume new functional roles. This is the essence of the qualitative changes associated with stage transitions in organismic theory [*Pinard and Laurendeau,* 1969; *Werner,* 1957; *Werner and Kaplan,* 1963] and exemplified in the changing relationships among sensory-motor-perceptual and logico-symbolic functioning across the human life span. Increased differentiation (the additivity and specificity assumption) is always accompanied by a concomitant increase in hierarchic integration [*Werner,* 1957]. What this means in behavioral terms, of course, is that lower-level response modes such as the perceptual assume qualitatively different functional salience after higher-level potentials such as the symbolic are attained. This does not deny the possibility that earlier dominant response categories may continue to evidence progressive development during later stages and may indeed become temporarily characteristic during periods of stress or functional disruption [*Flavell,* 1971, 1977; *Langer,* 1970]. This leads to major problems in diagnosing an individual as belonging in any developmental stage. It makes somewhat problematical the developmental synchrony or 'abruptness' assumptions usually associated with Piagetian stage transitions. However, some recent writers have questioned the logical necessity of such assumptions in the Piagetian system [*Feldman and Toulmin,* 1976; *Flavell,* 1970, 1971, 1977]. [*F. Hooper,* 1979, p. 142.]

The question now remains: To what extent do the family developmental cycles or stages discussed by *Hill and Mattessich* [1979] meet these rather stringent criteria set by the organicists? One must remember that developmental change is an a priori assumption of organismic theory, not a derived term or state of affairs as viewed by the mechanistic writers (in parallel with the distinction between quantum versus classical Newtonian physics where relative movement rather than static states is assumed as given). In brief, an external force is *not* absolutely necessary and sufficient to move the organism or system along its developmental path. Rather, the individual and its larger systems (including the family locus?) provides its *own* impetus for developmental progression and possible regression. One must also bear in mind that according to organismic theory quantitative increments in one domain may well result in qualitative leaps in a corollary behavioral dimension. Certainly the converse is also true, for qualitative changes often permit major quantitative increments in similar or related response categories.

While an entire chapter could be devoted to the issue of terminology usage and confusion between family and individual developmental theories, one clue to whether *Hill and Mattessich* [1979, pp. 173–174] really adhere to qualitative alterations across the family stages is their treatment of two key terms, structural differentiation and related transformations. As described above, structural characteristics, integration, and the associated qualitative transformations are certainly critical concepts for *Piaget* and *Werner*. For *Hill and Mattessich* [1979], significant structural change appears to involve the introduction of three factors, i.e., the number of persons in the family complex, their respective role assignments, and the associated patterns of roles and other interactive or transactive behavior present at a given point in family time. They comment that 'The concept of "related transformations" implies that the family moves from one stage to the next, restructuring its pattern of organization, yet with common threads tying all stages together' [p. 174]. In this context they cite the game-tree model of *Magrabi and Marshall* [1965] as representative of the family's movement along potentially alternative developmental pathways to similar outcomes. We are simply not sure if this family development model demands the same stringent criteria as those put forth by *Piaget* and *Werner* regarding stage characteristics and associated transition variables.

The Relevance of Werner's Developmental Approach

As the reader may have surmised, we feel that one possibility for genuine rapprochement between individual and family theories of development across the life span lies in the theory and research of *Werner* [cf. *Glick*, 1982; *Pea*, 1982]. For example, *Werner's* [1957, p. 126] definition of development (the orthogenetic principle) is as follows:

> Developmental psychology postulates one regulative principle of development; it is an orthogenetic principle which states that wherever development occurs it proceeds from a state of relative globality and lack of differentiation to a state of increasing differentiation, articulation, and hierarchic integration.

There are a number of interesting points which follow from this approach to defining a valid developmental event. First, the central issue involves an immanent dialectic, i.e., 'how does a developing organism (or family system) change qualitatively and at the same time preserve its integrity?' [*Langer,* 1970, p. 733]. It is the paradox of developing systems that certain aspects of stability and continuity must coexist with adaptive changes. Thus, if one were to focus upon changes exclusively, fully half of the overall picture would be lost or at least obscured. Surely this is true of growth of the family system over its life span. Certain stability-maintaining functions must be present for the family to preserve its unique integrity whether viewed as the family of ego or as the lineage family [*Feldman and Feldman,* 1975]. There is, therefore, a microlevel dialectical process constantly in operation – increased differentiation and specialization – which in the family system leads to greater role and task complexity which should be balanced by increased hierarchic integration. In addition, as is true of all organic systems in disequilibrium, the family must ultimately secure external resources in an energy transfer sense [*Brent,* 1978], or face eventual *dis*organization and disintegration. This would appear to be especially important when internal family conflict is high and when external perturbations are increasing.

Another major consequence of the Wernerian view of development concerns the time dimension. One may note that time, per se, is not even mentioned in the definition. This 'timeless' view of developmental phenomena has certain major conceptual and empirical advantages. Since a finite time frame is not specified, the development of individuals and larger systems, which may contain the individual units, may be compared through formal analysis.

In this regard, it seems to us that the family development model, at least as it has been used by some proponents, has been inordinately 'time bound'. So many of the within-stage characteristics and across-stage transition processes appear to be tied to the duration of the marriage, the chronological ages of the participants, and the gain or loss of participants. One possible outcome of this preoccupation with the linear time variable may be a lack of appreciation for stage or cycle 'mixtures'; that is, the family may well function as if it were located in more than one stage for rather protracted developmental intervals.

Werner's comparative/organismic approach specifically provides for the possibility of bidirectional developmental changes of both a short-term nature (via the principle of genetic spirality) and in terms of longer-range processes (for example, *de*differentiation and consequent losses in integration in the typical aging phenomena). Thus it can be related to the curvilinearity assumptions of the family life cycle [see *Hill and Mattessich,* 1979, point 3, p. 199]. Although the *empirical* validity of certain curvilinear developmental trends has recently been questioned [e.g., see *Hudson and Murphy,* 1980, and *Spanier* et al., 1979, on marital adjustment], the *conceptual* status of these patterns appears to be well established for general organismic theory and family developmental theory.

A number of these attempts to assess the putative curvilinear relationship between family life cycle location and marital satisfaction indices appear decidedly simplistic in terms of research design and associated data analyses [*Hudson and Murphy,* 1980]. Thus in some cases ordinal stage locations have been correlated with interval scale marital satisfaction scores, and few investigators have employed trend analyses with orthogonal components permitting the exclusion or statistical adjustment of significant linear components in the resultant data sets.

These methodological caveats notwithstanding, the essential conceptual point appears to be missed by these writers. Applying quantitative linear statistical methods, which assume essential additivity of main effects and interaction values, albeit to a presumed higher-order component, represents a mechanistic corollary being imposed upon qualitatively discontinuous, nonadditive stage phenomena [*Overton and Reese,* 1973, pp. 82–84]. Thus the formal truth criteria of one world view (the mechanistic) are employed to evaluate the empirical validity of the counterpart organismic model. To the extent that family life-cycle stages or levels represent organized complexity rather than linear additivity this methodological model mixing is not justified. Moreover, *Hill* and his associates have never advocated a simple juxtaposition of chronological age or marriage duration for life cycle location vis-à-vis marital satisfaction outcomes. Sweeping pejoratives concerning possible type I errors in earlier research [*Hudson and Murphy,* 1980] and consequent doubts concerning the viability of the family life-cycle model as a research heuristic appear misguided or at least premature. This would certainly seem to be the case for the *Hudson and Murphy* [1980] data in which the youngest subjects were 40 years of age! Methodological rigor alone is a rather poor alternative to conceptual clarity in translating a model's logical outcomes into valid research designs.

For *Hill and Mattessich* [1979], the concepts of chronological versus logical (structural) analysis appear to be confused. The particular nature of the family structure and its subsequent alterations (whether progressive/regressive or functional/dysfunctional) are not necessarily tied to chronological time except in the most trivial sense. Thus the major problems regarding stage transitions and continuity versus discontinuity of changes across the family cycle [*Hill and Mattessich,* 1979, pp. 181–182] become pseudoproblems from the view of *structural time* [*Overton and Reese,* 1981, pp. 114–117; *Werner,* 1957, p. 133]. This permits the investigator to deal with stage mixtures, multiple-level functioning, and potentially dysfunctional movement within the family system under stress. [For a recent example of the latter situation as posed in structural terms, see *Hoffman,* 1980, or *Olson* et al., 1979.]

Of course, it is possible that *Hill and Mattessich* do not really subscribe to the more stringent assumptions and corollary outcomes of organismic theory. Thus, they quote *Aldous* [1975, p. 102]:

> To save ourselves from being misunderstood we should emphasize that our use of the term *stage* does not imply that these stages are invariant, irreversible, or always occur in this order, properties that the stage concept has when it is used to refer to the development of organisms. The listed stages are neither prescriptive nor descriptive of all family life cycles. Since there is no rigid chronological sequence of events, multiple variations of stages are possible within the general overall sequence.

They further conclude, '... Our targets for explanation are moving targets rather than 'stages' or 'products': multidirectional paths of development which depart from the usual unidirectional linear models; and reversible, recursive relations among the indicators of family development' [*Hill and Mattessich,* 1979, p. 200]. Whatever the family stages or cycles really are for *Hill and Mattessich,* they are evidently *not* the type of structural entities used by *Piaget.* Perhaps they are closer to the concept of levels as formulated by *Werner* [*Glaserfeld and Kelly,* 1982; *Glick,* 1982].

By way of summary, *Werner's* approach is expressed in three related ideas [*Langer,* 1970]. First, *discontinuity* is provided through the differentiation process whereby a relatively global organization becomes a more individuated whole. Secondly, *continuity* is provided via the construct of hierarchic integration. 'As a consequence, some forms of the organism's structures and functions are preserved by being subsumed by the more individual systems that have developed; not all primitive systems are lost or altered in the course of developing competence' [*Langer,* 1970, p. 735]. This leads to the possibility of multilevel functioning during the mature years [*Kramer,* 1983; *Labouvie-Vief,* 1980, 1982] and should be equally applicable to the multiple functioning capacities of family systems over their life course (might not earlier stage-specific functioning reappear, albeit in altered form, at more advanced stages of family development?). Finally, a dialectical *synthesis* of the above components is provided for by *Werner.*

The organization of a new stage is a reorganization of the previous stage that combines both continuity and discontinuity. The total pattern is altered but still continuous with the previous pattern: (a) new structures and functions are dominant and hierarchically integrate or control others; (b) differentiation leads to specialization and newly individuated systems, and (c) primitive systems that are preserved operate differently due to increased centralization and their regulation by more differentiated and integrated systems [*Langer,* 1970, p. 735].

Thus, *Werner's* general approach and specific definitions appear to provide an ideal vehicle for integrating individual developmental patterns within larger social units such as the family system and the cohort-specific generational milieu. If these larger units also display the fundamental differentiation and integration attributes described above, they also qualify as genuine developmental phenomena. We feel that this is indeed the case and, further, that these considerations are particularly germane to subsequent revisions of the family developmental model.

Family Developmental Theory: Some Questions

Individual development theorists have been concerned about the use of various constructs as descriptive versus explanatory versus predictive [e.g., *Baltes* et al., 1977; *Brainerd,* 1978, 1979]. Similarly, we feel it is important that theorists working with family development theory answer the question, How is the theory to be used? *Hill and Mattessich* [1977] have urged 'reworking the taxonomy of concepts for *describing* and the emergent theories for *explaining* the phenomena of family development' [p. 5, emphases added] and have asserted that 'the sequence of variations in family organization is a *predictable* sequence which can be, and has been, identified through family research' [p. 9, emphasis added]. Thus, it would appear that family development is describable, predictable, and susceptible to explanation. However, a careful reading of the *Hill and Mattessich* [1977] paper reveals a somewhat indiscriminate use of the term 'family development' to cover all three cases. As with individual development, the danger lies in falling into tautological reasoning: Family development is seen to be occurring because the family is developing, and we can therefore predict that development will continue. Researchers and theorists using the family development approach must observe the fundamental principle of 'a priori dichotomization of data' [*Coombs* et al., 1954]. That is, the original data which inspired the theory can in no way be used to validate the theory in question [cf. *Brainerd,* 1981, p. 66]. *Hill and Mattessich* [1979, p. 200] have

noted that the ultimate goal of family development theorists is 'the generation of two types of substantive theory: (1) theories of the phenomenon of
family development, and (2) an improved family development theory of the
economic and social achievements of families. The first makes variety in
life-span family development the consequent or dependent variable to be
explained. The second makes "family development" the antecedent or
determinant variable in a cause-effect sequence model'. As *Kaplan* [1967,
p. 81] has pointed out, 'every key "catchword" has been invested with multiple, and sometimes even antithetical meanings, not only in different theories, but in what is presumably the same theory. "Development" is clearly
such a catchword'.

A central question may thus be posed: Will family development theorists and researchers use the term 'family development' to describe, explain,
or predict, or all of these, and how will the distinctions be kept clear? The
theoretical categories or objectives of description versus explanation versus
prediction are inevitably arbitrary and, indeed, can only be viewed as separate epistemological endeavors in an abstract manner [*Kaplan,* 1964; *Sigel,*
1979; *White,* 1978]. Ideally, these categories blend into one another in order
to produce a greater understanding of the human condition. Excluding radical behaviorists [*Zuriff,* 1980], the usual order of affairs demands descriptive observations as precursors of explanatory constructs and predictive
relationships. To the present writers it appears heuristically convenient to
consider explanatory variables and related hypothetical constructs as the
obvious products of theory builders such as *Hill,* and expedient to relegate
prediction problems to the area of external validity and scope. While we
realize that the inherent world view [*F. Hooper,* 1973; *Overton and Reese,*
1973] or spatiotemporal position [*Heisenberg,* 1958] of the observer may
indeed serve to bias the initial observations at issue, the essential first-order
task is the descriptive endeavor. Following this collection of normative
data, the explanatory and predictive functions feed back upon each other
and serve to also modify the original descriptive base. The final objective of
these endeavors is the specification of causal relationships among antecedent, concurrent (including structural determinants), and consequent variables as these factors influence the developing individual and family across
the life span [*Baltes* et al., 1980].

Another aspect of family development about which similar questions
may be raised is the use of the role concept. *Jackson* [1970, pp. 127–128]
argued the 'inseparability of the role concept from a culture-limited view of
family structure', and noted that:

There is no clear line between the role as descriptive or as idealistic; that is, people are classified by conformity or nonconformity to predetermined categories which are products either of cultural stereotype or theoretical bias. The implication is that the healthy family has Father in the father role, Mother in the mother role, Son in the male child role, etc. ... A role, with its theoretically concomitant behaviors, exists independently of behavioral data. That is, not only the general notion of role, but the specifics of the various sorts of family roles are theoretical, not phenomenological. When observational data is [sic] involved, it is in relation to the theoretical role as model ('inadequate performance of a role', 'role break-down', 'role reversal'). It seems apparent that analysis of such discrepancies between model and reality only emphasizes further the gap between categories and data.

While *Jackson's* was an admittedly conservative view of the applicability of role theory to the family case, he did raise some provocative questions with which family development theory will need to grapple. How will the theory avoid the trap of equating the role and its concomitant career with the role-taker? Why does an individual assume his or her respective role, and why does '... the internalization of the family role structure on the part of one child ... make him schizophrenic, but on the part of another child ... make him neurotic or even normal?' [*Meissner,* 1970, p. 157]. How, in more general terms, will researchers using a theoretical model which rests on role theory avoid making invidious comparisons from real families to the role model offered by the theory?

The theory builder may rightly protest that these questions come from clinicians whose interest in families is of a different sort and at a different level of analysis. However, we are suggesting that the ability of family development theory to address questions such as these may in the end determine its usefulness as a theory. We arbitrarily and randomly selected three issues of the *Journal of Marriage and the Family* and two issues of the *Family Coordinator* from our shelves and read the tables of contents. From this 'investigation', we found a large number of articles addressing questions similar to those raised by the clinicians noted above. For example, *Calonico and Thomas* [1973, p. 655] were inquiring into the question of whether 'role-taking is a function of the level of affect in interpersonal relationships together with the degree of similarity of value system'. In 1975, *Miller* was reporting on research designed to determine whether child spacing rather than child density might not be a more useful measure when investigating the effect of childbearing on marital satisfaction and conventionalization. *Movius* [1976, p.58] noted, in a provocative article on voluntary childlessness, that 'amazingly little research has been done on the motivation for parenthood'. *Clark* et al. [1978, p. 20] note that 'an understanding of time use in the work-family role system requires research on the allocation of time to *multiple* sectors and the place of individuals' preference structures in this process'. Finally, we found that *Marotz-Baden* et al. [1979, p. 5] were asserting, based on a review of literature on the effects of alternative family forms, that it is 'more fruitful to consider the social interaction dynamics that lead to a given outcome than to focus on the form of the family as the critical independent variable'.

One of us [*J. Hooper,* 1979a, b] has found, in a sample of families whose mother has returned to school as a university student, that what seems to be important to families is not role-taking behavior, but rather the perceived *meaning* of the behavior. Thus, a specific behavior, such as dishwashing by the husband, may be seen as supportive ['He's very helpful. He's even taken over the dishwashing.') in one family, and as nonsupportive in another family ('He's not helpful at all. It just about kills him that he has to do the dishes.').

All of these studies, and many others as well, lead us to the following question: If it should prove to be the case that the critical issues in family studies are not *what* families and family members do, nor *when* they do it, but rather *how,* and above all, *why* they do what they do, will family development theory have the ability to deal with these issues? We believe that to achieve explanatory power, family development theory will need to take account of inter- and intrafamily differences in such variables as belief systems, family history and myth, and the meanings of roles and role-taking; in short, we believe family development theory must deal with what *Kantor and Lehr* [1975] have called the interior of the family. Indeed, it seems to us that *Hill and Mattessich* [1979, p. 173] have noted this same need:

> We need a working definition of family development which reflects change in the family ... as well as changes in the personalities of individual members ... Changes in interpersonal relationships, in dyadic and triadic attachments, in the building and breaking of family bonds, and in family cultural orientations deserve analysis in their own right as families change in form and function over their life span.

The Issue of External Validity

It is obvious that family development theory, as all theories, reflects the world views and values of the theory builders [*Gouldner,* 1970]. At the least, these theorists believe that families consist of a married man and woman and at least one child. In addition, the theory, as it is presently formulated, deals with such families only so long as they remain intact, the termination point of the family occurring at the death (usually in old age) of one of the marital pair. Certainly the theorists may choose to deal with only those families which progress through the specified sequence, although the critic may then justifiably inquire about the value of a theory which deals with a limited proportion of the population of families. This leads us to the critical issue of external validity. There is no need to quote here the population data with which all of us are familiar [*Carter and Glick,* 1976; *Trost,* 1973]. Even acknowledging the operational complexities in defining comparison cohorts [e.g., *Nydegger,* 1981; *Rosow,* 1978], we submit that the number of families of which the sequence is descriptive becomes proportionally smaller year by year, and that this is not a trivial problem. We note that *Hill and Mattessich* [1979, p. 170] are aware of this problem: 'it (the theory) appears ... to have been exclusively oriented to the developmental cycle of [intact?] nuclear family units'. *Hill* [1979, p. 3] has noted that 'Uhlenberg and Glick both suggest that the modal nuclear family cycle was experienced by as high as 69% of cohorts born in the 1930s, higher than ever before in US history, and estimate that more than 50% will do so in the birth cohorts of the 1970s'. We would point out that these figures indicate an approximate 19% decline in persons experiencing the nuclear family cycle in only 40 years, and that the decline appears to be continuing, if not accelerating, into the 80s [Population Reference Bureau, 1982].

Hill and Mattessich [1977, p. 19] have also argued that 'the family actively manipulates its environment rather than being primarily acted upon by its environment'. To the extent that this statement is meant to refer to the near environment of a given family over its life span, we would not quibble. We feel, though, that family development theorists have a larger and longer field of vision in mind for the theory; certainly *Hill and Mattessich* [1979] acknowledge the additional power of the theory if it can be made to account for cultural and long-range historical variation. *Demos* [1977, p. 77] has argued compellingly that familial-societal processes move '*from* the society at large, *to* the family in particular', and he has commented that 'On the checkerboard of social institutions, the family seems to display a markedly reactive character. Time and again, it receives influences from without, rebuffs them, modifies them, adapts to them'. Similarly, *Norton* [1980, p. 68] has commented that 'measures of marital and family events are not only sensitive to subcultural factors but, also, in an overriding sense, to historical contingencies'. *Toffler* [1980, p. 211], in particular, has painted a vivid picture of the necessity for families to respond to vast changes in societies. He suggests that the nuclear family evolved in response to the industrial revolution, supplanting the 'extended family', in whatever form, of agricultural societies, and that a new 'Third Wave' society is causing 'not the death of the family as such, but the final fracture of the Second Wave (industrial) family system in which all families were supposed to emulate the idealized nuclear model, and the emergence in its place of a diversity of family forms'.

Thus, we believe that societal acceptance of behaviors such as divorcing and living together, as well as increasing stress on the nuclear family (inflation, energy shortages, expectations for personal fulfillment, the need for more than one income, intrusion by media, etc.) will combine to further decrease the number of families to which the theory applies. If one accepts this point of view, then the frequently noted homily 'there have always been nuclear families' loses its apparent predictive power; that is, the nuclear family with its typical life course sequence may, primarily as a result of larger societal changes, become a thing of the past.

Family Stage Transitions

Whether or not this possibility comes to pass, and leaving aside the consequences of such a possibility, *today's* reality forcibly suggests that family development theory has so far failed to deal effectively with the more interesting, and possibly more profitable, points of transition in family life cycles. Recent evidence from a methodological study by *Spanier* et al. [1979, p. 37] suggests that the identification of transition points could lead to a specification of stage boundaries. They note that this approach 'may yield more relevant developmental stages than the usual family life cycle stages'.

There have, of course, been attempts to conceptualize theoretical and research models of transition points. The previously mentioned *Magrabi and Marshall* [1965] game-tree model for the study of alternate pathways also dealt with family transitions. *Burr* [1972] created the concept 'ease of transition' to account for the variability among families in a given stage, and in a family from one stage to another; some families have rough and others smooth changes in structure from stage to stage. *Klein* and his colleagues [*Borne* et al., 1979; *Klein* et al., 1977] have discussed the Duvall-Hill model [*Duvall,* 1971], characterizing it as stage discrete, such that different scores on variables of interest would be obtained from modal families in adjacent stages. In contrast, the *Rapoport* [1963] model, which *Klein* called 'stage-transitional', makes the transitions the major point of interest. As *Klein* has noted, the Duvall-Hill model does not address this issue, while the Rapoport model disregards questions about differences between families before or after transitions. *Klein* and his colleagues offered a third model which combines the previous two, and adds the concept that there may be intrafamilial differences preceding the following transitions.

It should be noted that the transitions across Piagetian stages, for example, have not been clearly elaborated either. As early as 1962, *Kessen* identified this as a major problem within stage-specific Piagetian theory. This problem remains a preoccupation of both the Genevan and other neo-Piagetian writers [e.g., *Campbell and Richie*, 1983; *Feldman and Toulmin*, 1976; *Overton and Reese*, 1981]. Piaget, in his later years, became particularly concerned with the processes which underlie stage movement and change. This included an interest in such diverse topics as motivational factors, learning and socialization processes, and conscious awareness as related to alterations in psychological structure [e.g., *Bringuier*, 1980; *Piaget*, 1976, 1978, 1981; *Piatelli-Palmarini*, 1980].

In similar fashion, we believe that the family development theory of the future will most likely include a focus upon the critical stage-transition process. That is, although the family development theory, as presently formulated, adequately describes the life-cycle stages of a number of families, the task remains for family development theory to be able to encompass alternative sequences *and* to explain the critical transition points at which families move in other directions. The formulations of *Klein* and his colleagues appear to be moving in that direction.

Conclusions

It appears that many of the problems of family development theory stem from a tendency among both adherents and critics to combine levels of analysis. This may be best viewed as a metatheoretical problem. In terms of both causal complexity and distal/proximal relations, the family, as a structural entity, lies at an intermediate level between individual growth and development patterns and larger societal institutions [*Bengtson*, 1977]. Thus, families as research or theory targets have either macro-characteristics or micro-characteristics, depending upon the perspective of the initial observation. Since we agree with *Kaplan* [1967] and *Riegel* [1976] that no single level of analysis can be accorded primary status, it follows that observers of both family and individual development must acknowledge the possibility of causal interconnections across the levels of analysis typically emphasized. One particularly useful way to view the levels of analysis is to consider the respective time frames. Development from an individual perspective includes processes which range from microseconds at the cellular level to intergenerational changes and continuities. The major institutions of a given society or culture are generally viewed in an even longer time range, although shorter-term stabilities and alteration processes are also of interest.

From the present perspective, the individual family unit may be seen as occupying a central focus which shares each of these temporal orientations; its development is probably a complex outcome of forces originating at both the individual and larger societal levels. The importance of the global time frame embodying historico-cultural contexts for individual development [*Baltes* et al., 1980; *Labouvie-Vief and Chandler*, 1978; *Riegel*, 1976], and sociological analyses, including the family case [*Elder*, 1977; *Featherman*, 1983], were considered by *Hill and Mattessich* [1979, pp. 190–191]. Indeed, it should be pointed out that a number of the issues discussed in the present chapter are covered to varying degrees by *Hill and Mattessich* [1979]. These include levels of analysis and associated time dimensions [pp. 190–191], historical contexts and cohort-specific discontinuities [pp. 192–194], the general issue of universality versus relativity of family developmental patterns [pp. 195–197], and a series of suggested new dimensions designed to increase the descriptive accuracy and potential explanatory power of family development theory [pp. 197–200]. The actual implementation of these constructs within family development theory, however, remains to be accomplished.

Insofar as individual development is concerned, attempts have been made to relate differing levels of analysis (e.g., the biological and the psychological) to the presence of additivity versus nonadditivity, continuity versus discontinuity, emergent versus nonnovel events, and the general issue of quantitative versus qualitative change across the life span [cf. *Nydegger*, 1981, pp. 21–22; *Werner*, 1957, pp. 133–137; see also *Brent*, 1985; *Lerner*, 1978; *Overton and Reese*, 1981]. Many of these efforts [see especially *Nagel*, 1957] tacitly assume a completely deterministic world view; that is, what is left unexplained at one level will eventually be linked to causal relationships at a different level of analysis.

The major problem here, of course, lies in the fact that many systems of interest are governed by causal laws only in a *probabilistic* sense both in the inorganic physical case [*Heisenberg,* 1959; *Pais,* 1982] and in developing organisms [*Labouvie-Vief,* 1975; *Mayr,* 1982] and large areas of statistical uncertainty remain. Judging by examples in particle and quantum physics (which many behavioral scientists are wont to imitate [cf. *Datan,* 1977], the areas of statistical indeterminancy may be nonoverlapping between the levels of analysis, thus necessitating mutually exclusive yet complementary theoretical models for a given range of developmental events [*Heisenberg,* 1958; *Overton,* 1983; *Pais,* 1982]. Perhaps the most ambitious recent attempt to identify the possible causal influences on individual development in a life-span context is that of *Baltes* et al. [1980]. They distinguish three categories of interactive influences, normative age-graded (e.g., biological and biogenetic factors), normative history-graded (e.g., current socioenvironmental factors), and nonnormative life events (e.g., '...antecedent patterns associated with career changes, relocation, medical traumata, accidents, temporary unemployment, divorce, institutionalization, and the death of significant others', p. 76). Hypothetical life-course profiles which reflect the varying degrees of influence are then presented.

In the context of micro- versus macro-processes [*Bengtson,* 1977], certain questions remain unanswered when the general levels-of-analysis approach is applied to the family development case. Are the modes of explanation or the types of causation (as discussed earlier) dependent upon the levels of analysis selected? Are the same (identical versus isomorphically parallel) causal relationships which are found to hold for one level likely to be found at the counterpart levels? And finally, what conceptual and/or empirical confounding may be produced by a nondiscriminate mixing of our levels of analysis? A clear conceptual separation of the microlevel and macrolevel influences within a general causal matrix is equally important for the family and individual developmental cases.

Piaget's structural approach represents only one way of dealing with the interrelations among differing levels, in this case the biological, psychological, and sociological realms of individual development. Nonetheless, his comments are most instructive:

In this sense, society is the supreme unit, and the individual can only achieve his inventions and intellectual constructions insofar as he is the seat of collective interactions that are naturally dependent, in level and value, on society as a whole ... society is nevertheless a product of life ... So the important question is not how to assess the respective merits of individual and group ... but to see the logic in solitary reflection as in cooperation, and to see the errors and follies both in collective opinion and individual conscience [*Piaget,* 1971, p. 368].

The complexities and differing viewpoints of the literature cited in the present chapter lead one to believe that a genuine rapprochement of the family and individual developmental theorists will be a difficult undertaking. However, an eventual blending of the two theory and research areas is essential to a more complete understanding of the individual and the family. The recent efforts of *Hill and Mattessich* [1979] and others [e.g., *Bengtson and Dowd,* 1980/81; *Featherman,* 1983; *Gadlin,* 1980; *Hartup,* 1978; *Reid,* 1984] must be evaluated as essential first steps approaching this problem.

From our perspective, much of what *Hill and Mattessich* [1977, 1979] have attempted in reconstructing family development theory vis-à-vis information from disparate disciplines is essentially similar to the efforts of dialectics/systems and contextualist writers in the individual development domain [e.g., *Labouvie-Vief and Chandler,* 1978; *Overton,* 1983; *Riegel,* 1976; *Tolman,* 1981]. Also in similar fashion the result is not a novel theory as such, for many of the essential features of formal theory construction, such as logically derived principles, postulates, and empirically testable assumptions, are lacking [*Hage,* 1972]. Rather, the present family development theory, as is true of the dialectics/systems approach, is best viewed as a model or metatheory [*Reid,* 1984] which can serve to heuristically guide family scholars.

As *Holman and Burr* [1980, p. 734] noted,

> The general theories that are useful in understanding family phemomena deal with different aspects of a very complex subject area, and we cannot even envision what a unifying perspective would be like. It would have to include such diverse concerns as economic, social, biological, physical, aesthetic, spiritual, psychological, historical, and governmental factors. As a result, it would have to be either extremely massive so that all of the factors could be included at a reasonable level of generality or so oversimplifying that it would provide little information about these complex phenomena. We suspect that the pattern that presently exists is probably the most effective one for family theories. Therefore, we ought to quit looking for a theory that will provide 'overarching underpinnings'.

Thus, the family development approach may ultimately function as a model which will serve to help family scholars remain aware of the complexities of family functioning, and the dangers of simplistic thinking about families, while they investigate manageable questions. From our point of view, the family development approach represents a significant improvement upon earlier static structure-function models. By highlighting the dynamic aspects of *developing* families in a changing environment, the family development approach has brought new impetus to the field of family and individual studies.

Acknowledgements

This is an extended revision of a paper presented at the Theory Construction and Research Methodology Workshop of the Annual Meeting of the National Council on Family Relations, Boston, Mass. The authors acknowledge the helpful comments of their colleagues: *Pauline G. Boss,* University of Minnesota; *James E. Johnson,* Pennsylvania State University, and *Ronald M. Sabatelli,* University of Connecticut; and the workshop discussants: *Erik Felsinger,* Arizona State University, and especially *Reuben Hill,* University of Minnesota.

References

Aldous, J.: The developmental approach to family analysis. Unpublished manuscript (University of Georgia, Athens 1975).

Baltes, P.B.; Reese, H.W.; Lipsitt, L.P.: Life-span developmental psychology; in Rosenzweig, Porter, Annual review of psychology (Annual Reviews, Palo Alto 1980).

Baltes, P.B.; Reese, H.W.; Nesselroade, J.R.: Life-span developmental psychology: introduction to research methods (Books/Cole, Monterey 1977).

Beilin, H.: Learning and operational convergence in logical thought development. J. exp. Child Psychol. *2:* 317–339 (1965).

Beilin, H.: Developmental stages and developmental processes; in Ross, Ford, Flamer, Measurement and Piaget (McGraw-Hill, New York 1971).

Beilin, H.: Research programs and revolutions in developmental psychology. Symp. Bienn. Meet. Soc. Res. Child Dev., Detroit 1983.

Bengtson, V.: Reconstruction of family development theory: an exercise in the study of micro-social organization through time. Theory Construction and Research Methodology Workshop, National Council on Family Relations Annual Meeting, San Diego 1977.

Bengtson, V.L.; Dowd, J.J.: Sociological functionalism, exchange theory, and life-cycle analysis: a call for more explicit theoretical bridges. Int. J. Aging hum. Dev. *12:* 55–73 (1980/81).

Bickhard, M.H.: The nature of developmental stages. Hum. Dev. *21:* 217–233 (1978).

Bijou, S.W.; Baer, D.M.: Child development, vol. 1: A systematic and empirical theory (Appleton, New York 1961).

Borne, H.; Jacke, A.; Sederberg, N.; Klein, D.M.: Family chronogram analysis: toward the development of new methodological tools for assessing the life cycles of families. Theory Construction and Research Methodology Workshop, National Council on Family Relations Annual Meeting, Boston 1979.

Braine, M.D.S.: The ontogeny of certain logical operations: Piaget's formulation examined by nonverbal methods. Psychol. Monogr. *73:* 475 (1959).

Brainerd, C.J.: The stage question in cognitive developmental theory. Behav. Brain Sci. *2:* 173–182 (1978).

Brainerd, C.J.: Continuing commentary on the stage question in cognitive-developmental theory. Behav. Brain Sci. *2:* 137–154 (1979).

Brainerd, C.J.: Stage II: a review of 'Beyond universals in cognitive development'. Devl. Rev. *1:* 63–81 (1981).

Brent, S.B.: Prigogine's model for self-organization in nonequilibrium systems: its relevance for developmental psychology. Hum. Dev. *21:* 374–387 (1978).

Brent, S.: Psychological structures and their functions: a morphogenetic approach (Springer, New York 1985).

Bringuier, J.: Conversations with Jean Piaget (University of Chicago Press, Chicago 1980).

Bruner, J.S.: The course of cognitive growth. Am. Psychol. *19:* 1–15 (1964).

Burr, W.R.: Role-transitions: a reformulation of theory. J. Marr. Fam. *34:* 407–416 (1972).

Calonico, J.M.; Thomas, D.L.: Role-taking as a function of value similarity and affect in the nuclear family. J. Marr. Fam. *35:* 655–665 (1973).

Campbell, D.T.: Factors related to the validity of experiments in social settings. Psychol. Bull. *54:* 297–312 (1957).

Campbell, D.T.; Stanley, J.C.: Experimental and quasi-experimental designs for research; in Gage, Handbook of research on teaching (Rand McNally, Chicago 1963).

Carter, H.; Glick, P.: Marriage and divorce: a social and economic study (rev. ed.). Vital and Health Statistics Monographs, American Public Health Association (Harvard University Press, Cambridge 1976).

Chandler, M.J.: Relativism and the problem of epistemological loneliness. Hum. Dev. *18:* 171–180 (1975).

Clark, R.A.; Nye, F.I.; Gecas, V.: Husbands' work involvement and marital role performance. J. Marr. Fam. *40:* 9–21 (1978).

Cook, T.D.; Campbell, D.T.: Quasi-experimentation: design and analysis issues for field settings (Rand McNally, Chicago 1979).

Coombs, C.H.; Raiffia, H.; Thrall, R.M.: Some views of mathematical models and measurement theory. Psychol. Rev. *61:* 132–144 (1954).

Datan, N.: After the apple: post-Newtonian physics for jaded psychologists; in Datan, Reese, Life-span developmental psychology: dialectical perspectives on experimental research (Academic Press, New York 1977).

Demos, J.: The American family in past time; in Skolnick, Skolnick, Family in transition; 2nd ed. (Little, Brown, New York 1977).

Duvall, E.M.: Family development; 4th ed. (Lippincott, New York 1971).

Edelman, M.W.: Who is for children? Am. Psychol. *36:* 109–116 (1981).

Edelstein, W.; Noam, G.: Regulatory structures of the self and 'postformal' stages in adulthood. Hum. Dev. *25:* 407–422 (1982).

Elder, G.H.: Family history and the life course. J. Fam. History *2:* 279–304 (1977).

Featherman, D.L.: The life-span perspective in social science research; in Baltes, Brim, Life-span development and behavior, vol. 5 (Academic Press, New York 1983).

Feldman, C.F.; Toulmin, S.: Logic and the theory of mind; in Arnold, Nebraska symposium on motivation 1975: conceptual foundations of psychology (University of Nebraska Press, Lincoln 1976).

Feldman, H.; Feldman, M.: The family life cycle: some suggestions for recycling. J. Marr. Fam. *37:* 277–284 (1975).

Flavell, J.H.: Concept development; in Mussen, Carmichael's manual of child psychology, vol. 1 (Wiley, New York 1970).

Flavell, J.H.: Stage-related properties of cognitive development. Cognitive Psychol. *2:* 421–453 (1971).

Flavell, J.H.: Cognitive development (Prentice-Hall, Englewood Cliffs 1977).

Flavell, J.H.: Structures, stages, and sequences in cognitive development; in Collins, Minnesota Symposium in Child Psychology, vol. 15 (Erlbaum, Hillsdale 1981).

Flavell, J.H.: On cognitive development. Child Dev. *53:* 1–10 (1982).

Gadlin, H.: Dialectics and family interaction. Hum. Dev. *23:* 245–253 (1980).

Gagné, R.M.: Contributions of learning to human development. Psychol. Rev. *75:* 177–191 (1968).

Glaserfeld, E.; Kelly, M.F.: On the concepts of period, phase, stage, and level. Hum. Dev. *25:* 152–160 (1982).

Glick, J.: Heinz Werner's significance for contemporary developmental theory. Am. Psychol. Ass., Div. 7 Newsl. 18–23 (Washington, D.C. 1982).

Gouldner, A.W.: The coming crisis in Western sociology (Avon Books, New York 1970).

Hage, J.: Techniques and problems of theory construction in sociology (Wiley, New York 1972).

Hartup, W.: Perspectives on child and family interaction: past, present, and future; in Lerner, Spanier, Child influences on marital and family interaction: a life-span perspective (Academic Press, New York 1978).

Heisenberg, W.: The physicist's conception of nature (Harcourt, Brace & World, New York 1958).

Heisenberg, W.: Physik und Philosophie (Hirzel, Stuttgart 1959).

Hill, R.: Theories and research designs linking family behavior and child development: a critical overview. 16th International Family Research Seminar on the Child and the Family, St. Paul 1979.

Hill, R.; Mattessich, P.: Reconstruction of family development theories: a progress report. Theory Construction and Research Methodology Workshop, National Council on Family Relations Annual Meeting, San Diego 1977.

Hill, R.; Mattessich, P.: Family development theory and life-span development; in Baltes, Brim, Life-span development and behavior, vol. 2 (Academic Press, New York 1979).

Hill, R.; Rodgers, R.H.: The developmental approach; in Christensen, Handbook of marriage and the family (Rand McNally, Chicago 1964).

Hoffman, L.: The family life cycle and discontinous change; in Carter, McGoldrick, The family life cycle: a framework for family therapy, pp. 53–63 (Gardner Press, New York 1980).

Hollos, M.: Logical operations and role-taking abilities in two cultures: Norway and Hungary. Child Dev. *46:* 638–649 (1975).

Hollos, M.; Cowan, P.A.: Social isolation and cognitive development: logical operations and role-taking abilities in the three Norwegian settings. Child Dev. *44:* 630–641 (1973).

Holman, T.B.; Burr, W.: Beyond the beyond: the growth of family theories in the 1970s. J. Marr. Fam. *42:* 729–741 (1980).

Hooper, F.H.: Cognitive assessment across the life-span: methodological implications of the organismic approach; in Nesselroade, Reese, Life-span developmental psychology: methodological issues (Academic Press, New York 1973).

Hooper, F.H.: Brainerd on the cognitive structure and integration criteria. Behav. Brain Sci. *1:* 142–143 (1979).

Hooper, J.O.: My wife, the student. Fam. Coord. *28:* 459–471 (1979a).

Hooper, J.O.: Returning women students and their families: support and conflict. J. Coll. Student Personnel *20:* 145–152 (1979b).

Hudson, W.; Murphy, G.: The nonlinear relationship between marital satisfaction and stages of the family life cycle: an artifact of type I errors. J. Marr. Fam. *42:* 263–267 (1980).

Jackson, D.D.: The study of the family; in Ackerman, Family process (Basic Books, New York 1970).

Janik, A.; Toulmin, S.: Wittgenstein's Vienna (Simon & Schuster, New York 1973).

Kantor, D.; Lehr, W.: Inside the family: toward a theory of family process (Harper, New York 1975).

Kaplan, A.: The conduct of inquiry (Chandler, San Francisco 1964).

Kaplan, B.: Meditations on genesis. Hum. Dev. *10:* 65–87 (1967).

Kessen, W.: Stages and structure in the study of children. Monogr. Soc. Res. Child Dev. *27:* whole No. 103, pp. 65–86 (1962).

Klein, D.M.; Jorgensen, S.R.; Miller, B.C.: Methodological issues and strategies for assessing the influence of children on marital quality and family interaction over the life span. Unpublished manuscript. Pennsylvania State University Conference on Human and Family Development: Contributions of the child to marital quality and family interaction across the life span, State College, Pa., 1977.

Kramer, D.A.: Post-formal operations? A need for further conceptualization. Hum. Dev. *26:* 91–105 (1983).

Kreppner, K.; Paulsen, S.; Schuetze, Y.: Infant and family development: from triads to tetrads. Hum. Dev. *25:* 373–391 (1982).

Kurtines, W.M.: Measurability, description, and explanation: the explanatory adequacy of stage model. Behav. Brain. Sci. *2:* 192–194 (1978).

Labouvie, E.W.: The dialectical nature of measurement activities in the social sciences. Hum. Dev. *18:* 396–403 (1975).

Labouvie-Vief, G.: Beyond formal operations: uses and limits of pure logic in life-span development. Hum. Dev. *23:* 141–161 (1980).

Labouvie-Vief, G.: Dynamic development and mature autonomy: a theoretical prologue. Hum. Dev. *25:* 161–191 (1982).

Labouvie-Vief, G.; Chandler, M.J.: Cognitive development and life-span developmental theory: idealistic versus contextual perspectives; in Baltes, Life-span development and behavior, vol. 1 (Academic Press, New York 1979).

Lachman, R.: The model in theory construction. Psychol. Rev. *67:* 113–129 (1960).

Langer, J.: Werner's comparative organismic theory; in Mussen, Carmichael's manual of child psychology, vol. 1 (Wiley, New York 1970).

Lerner, R.: Nature, nurture, and dynamic interactionism. Hum. Dev. *21:* 1–20 (1978).

Looft, W.R.: Socialization and personality throughout the life-span: an examination of contemporary psychological approaches; in Baltes, Schaie, Life-span developmental psychology: personality and socialization (Academic Press, New York 1973).

Magrabi, F.M.; Marshall, W.H.: Family developmental tasks: a research model. J. Marr. Fam. *27:* 454–458 (1965).

Marotz-Baden, R.; Adams, G.; Bueche, N.; Munro, B.; Munro, G.: Family form or family process? Reconsidering the deficit family model approach. Fam. Coord. *28:* 5–14 (1979).

McGillicuddy, A.V.; Sigel, I.E.; Johnson, J.E.: The family as a system of mutual influences: parental beliefs, distancing behaviors, and children's representational thinking; in Lewis, Rosenblum, The child and his family (Plenum Press, New York 1979).

Mayr, E.: The growth of biological thought (Harvard University Press, Cambridge 1982).

Meissner, W.W.: Thinking about the family – psychiatric aspects; in Ackerman, Family process (Basic Books, New York 1970).

Merlino, F.J.: Metatheoretical isolationism reconsidered: its impact for developmental theories. Hum. Dev. *18:* 391–395 (1975).

Miller, B.C.: Child density, marital satisfaction, and conventionalization: a research note. J. Marr. Fam. *37:* 345–347 (1975).

Movius, M.: Voluntary childlessness: the ultimate liberation. Fam. Coord. *25:* 57–63 (1976).

Nagel, E.: Determinism and development; in Harris, The concept of development (University of Minnesota Press, Minneapolis 1957).

Norton, A.J.: The influence of divorce on traditional life-cycle measures. J. Marr. Fam. *42:* 63–69 (1980).

Olson, D.; Sprenkle, D.; Russel, C.: Circumplex model of marital and family systems. I. Cohesion and adaptability dimensions, family types, and clinical applications. Fam. Process *18:* 3–28 (1979).

Overton, W.F.: World views and their influence on psychological theory and research: Kuhn – Lakatos – Laudan; in Reese, Advances in child development and behavior (Academic Press, New York 1984).

Overton, W.F.; Reese, H.W.: Models of development: methodological implications; in Nesselroade, Reese, Life-span developmental psychology: methodological issues (Academic Press, New York 1973).

Overton, W.F.; Reese, H.W.: Conceptual prerequisites for an understanding of stability-change and continuity-discontinuity. Int. J. Behav. Dev. *4:* 99–123 (1981).

Page, R.C.; Smither, S.J.: Theory evaluation in developmental psychology: criticism of a popular view. Unpublished manuscript (University of Illinois, Champaign-Urbana).

Pais, A.: Max Born's statistical interpretation of quantum mechanics. Science *218:* 1193–1198 (1982).

Parish, T.S.; Parish, J.G.: Relationship between evaluation of one's self and one's own family by children from intact, reconstituted, and single-parent families. J. genet. Psychol. *143:* 293–294 (1983).

Pea, R.D.: Werner's influences on contemporary psychology. Hum. Dev. *25:* 303–308 (1982).

Pepper, S.C.: World hypotheses (University of California Press, Berkeley 1942).

Peterson, G.; Hey, R.; Peterson, L.: Intersection of family development and moral stage frameworks: implications for theory and research. J. Marr. Fam. *41:* 229–235 (1979).

Piaget, J.: The general problems of the psychobiological development of the child; in Tanner, Inhelder, Discussions on child development, vol. 4 (Tavistock, London 1960).

Piaget, J.: Piaget's theory; in Mussen, Carmichael's manual of child psychology, vol. 1 (Wiley, New York 1970).

Piaget, J.: Structuralism (Basic Books, New York 1970).

Piaget, J.: Biology and knowledge (University of Chicago Press, Chicago 1971).

Piaget, J.: Intellectual evolution from adolescence to adulthood. Hum. Dev. *12:* 1–12 (1972).

Piaget, J.: The grasp of consciousness (Harvard University Press, Cambridge 1976).

Piaget, J.: Success and understanding (Harvard University Press, Cambridge 1978).

Piaget, J.: Intelligence and affectivity: their relationship during child development (Annual Reviews, Palo Alto 1981).

Piatelli-Palmarini, M.: Language and learning: the debate between Jean Piaget and Noam Chomsky (Harvard University Press, Cambridge 1980).

Pinard, A.; Laurendeau, M.: 'Stage' in Piaget's cognitive-developmental theory: exegesis of a cocept; in Elkind, Flavell, Studies in cognitive development (Oxford University Press, New York 1969).

Population Reference Bureau: US Population: Where we are, where we're going (PRB, Washington 1982).

Rapoport, R.: Normal crises, family structure, and mental health. Fam. Processes *2:* 68–80 (1963).

Reese, H.W.; Overton, W.F.: Models of development and theories of development; in Goulet, Baltes, Life-span developmental psychology: research and theory (Academic Press, New York 1970).

Reid, B.V.: An anthropological reinterpretation of Kohlberg's stages of moral development. Hum. Dev. *27:* 57–64 (1984).

Riegel, K.F.: Dialectic operations: the final period of cognitive development. Hum. Dev. *16:* 346–370 (1973).

Riegel, K.F.: The dialectics of human development. Am. Psychol. *31:* 689–700 (1976).

Rosow, I.: What is a cohort and why? Hum. Dev. *21:* 65–75 (1978).

Segalen, M.: Research and discussion around family life cycle: an account of the 13th seminar on family research. J. Marr. Fam. *36:* 814–818 (1974).

Shantz, C.U.: A developmental study of Piaget's theory of logical multiplication. Merrill-Palmer Q. *13:* 121–137 (1967).

Sigel, I.E.: A structuralist response to a skeptic. Behav. Brain Sci. *2:* 148–149 (1979).

Spanier, G.B.; Lewis, R.A.; Cole, C.L.: Marital adjustment over the family life cycle: the issue of curvilinearity. J. Marr. Fam. *37:* 263–275 (1975).

Spanier, G.B.; Sauer, W.; Larzelere, R.: An empirical evaluation of the family life cycle. J. Marr. Fam. *41:* 27–38 (1979).

Toffler, A.: The third wave (Morrow, New York 1980).

Tolman, C.: The metaphysic of relations in Klaus Riegel's 'dialectics' of human development. Hum. Dev. *24:* 33–51 (1981).

Toulmin, S.: The concept of stages in psychological development; in Mischel, Cognitive development and epistemology, pp. 25–60 (Academic Press, New York 1971).

Trost, J.: The family life cycle: a problematic concept. 13th International Seminar on Family Research, International Sociological Association, Paris, France.

Waller, W.: The family: a dynamic interpretation (Cordon, New York 1938).

Werner, H.: The concept of development from a comparative and organismic point of view; in Harris, The concept of development (University of Minnesota Press, Minneapolis 1957).

Werner, H.; Kaplan, B.: Symbol formation (Wiley, New York 1963).

White, S.H.: Which comes first – describing or explaining? Behav. Brain Sci. 2: 205–206 (1978).

Wohlwill, J.F.: Piaget's system as a source of empirical research. Merrill-Palmer Q. 4: 253–262 (1963).

Wohlwill, J.F.: The study of behavioral development (Academic Press, New York 1973).

Zuriff, G.E.: Radical behaviorist epistemology. Psychol. Bull. 87: 337–350 (1980).

Contr. hum. Dev., vol. 14, pp. 31–60 (Karger, Basel 1985)

The Parental Imperative Revisited:
Towards a Developmental Psychology of
Adulthood and Later Life

David L. Gutmann

Northwestern University, Evanston, Ill., USA

When social scientists study aging in Western and urban settings, those in which older people are socially disadvantaged, they routinely discover that the second half of life is a period of escalating losses and depletions. In this catastrophic view, psychological development in later life is secondary, in reaction to primary losses, and comes about only when the aging person discovers adaptations which maintain the status quo and which temporarily hold disaster at bay. But those of us who have studied aging in more traditional folk societies, the natural gerontocracies, form a less gloomy picture of our human fate in the later years. In those settings, where the elders have the social leverage to arrange matters according to their own priorities, we find striking evidence of new development, new executive capacities of later life that go beyond mere adjustment to loss. Given such evidence, we think of the Third Age as a period marked by possibility of new growth as well as by the certainty of loss. In addition, since true development must, by definition, have a genetic base, we speculate about the evolutionary engines that could quicken new growth in the later years and about the purposes – species and social, as well as individual – served by these advances.

We know that adequate, 'good-enough' parenting is the necessary (if not sufficient) precondition for human development in the early years; and I have argued that the state of *parenthood,* of being parental, is a condition of equal force and dignity, powerful enough to drive the developmental transitions of adulthood, and even those of the later, postreproductive years. The remainder of this chapter will be devoted to fleshing out and justifying this large generalization.

The following points will be made: that the unique vulnerability of the human child requires a long period of parental service, such that parenthood is generally seen to be coextensive with adulthood; that parental assignments by gender are not an expression of male chauvinism, but are a response to the generic security requirements of helpless children; that the entry into the emergency condition of parenthood brings about a sharpening of sexual distinctions; that the phasing out of the parental emergency brings about a corresponding reduction in sex-role polarities, and a resumption of the prior, androgynous position on the part of both parents; and finally, that latent potentials, unused (because maladaptive) during parenthood, are released during the postparental years to bring about, under facilitating circumstances, the special developments that sustain species, society, and the individual during the later years.

Parenthood and Adulthood: An Identity

I have already argued [*Gutmann,* 1975] that parenthood should be understood from the generically human or species perspective, as the crucial organizer of human development in adult and later life, rather than from the more personal or idiosyncratic perspective (which defines parenthood as a potentially hedonic experience, to be 'consumed'). I held that parenthood and its associated activities represent the major junction points between the individual and the collective fate, the crucial status which ties individual satisfaction to universal, relatively invariant human goals. In this vein, I wrote: 'For most adult humans, parenthood is still the ultimate source of the sense of meaning. For most adults the question "What does life mean?" is automatically answered once they have children; better yet, it is no longer asked' [p. 170]. I added that: 'Transcultural regularities in sex-role training, in the male and female response to the "chronic emergency" of parenthood, and in the phasing out of parental responsibilities all suggest that sex distinctions have an intrinsic basis, and that they are organized around the vital requirements of young children. It is further argued that parenthood constitutes the pivotal stage of the human life cycle, organizing the form and content of the stages leading up to it, as well as those that succeed it. Accordingly, a study of the common denominators and requirements of human parenthood could be an important first step in developing a comparative psychology of the human life cycle' [p. 167].

We should keep in mind that the centrality of parenting in human (and primate) affairs is founded in paradox: It is an inescapable consequence of liberation, of the relative human freedom from inflexible instincts. Put bluntly, our infants are not born with a fixed behavioral repertoire, but instead with powerful cognitive and social *potentials*. This condition leaves them free to acquire new learning, but also terribly dependent for survival on the parent's good will and matured functions. In effect, the child's freedom to acquire new learning for itself – and ultimately for the entire species – binds that same child to a long childhood, and is solidly based on the adult's matching commitment to a long parental service. The bondage of the parental cohort is the evolutionary price that we pay for our species' relative freedom from instinctual coercion.

This dialectical relationship between infantile freedom and parental constraint is registered by most successful human groups in that they define a clear identity between mature adulthood and parenthood. Indeed, contemporary American society is one of the few in which a major attempt has been made (outside of monastic orders) to split adulthood from the parental condition. Most human societies are like the Kota of India, where *Mandelbaum* [1957] found that a Kota man does not think of himself as fully human until he has had children, 'until there is someone to call him father'. Similarly, *Levy* [1977], who studied adulthood among the Newars and in Tahiti, found at both sites that 'a responsible parenthood (the keeping and rearing of children) produces a shift in *informal social definition* to adulthood, confirming the earlier *ritual definition* at marriage'. And *Lowenthal* [1975], who studied the psychological effect of important life-span transitions, found that even in our relatively contraparental society 'family centeredness is a dominant theme in the protocols, and parenthood is the main transition envisaged by the young'.

Of course, and despite the family orientation of young adults, many individuals avoid parenthood; but this choice, made in young adulthood, may reveal its consequences only in later years. Thus, at Northwestern University Medical School, in our studies of late-onset psychiatric disorders, we find that childless older women are represented in the population of first-onset psychotics far beyond their representation in the population as a whole. Replicated in British and Scandinavian samples, these findings suggest that the childless state can have malignant consequences long after the original contraparental decision was first made. Like any other important motive, parenthood *can* be denied or repressed, but only at one's peril; the subjective will to denial does not negate the *objective* importance of the denied motive.

I became intuitively aware of the equation between adulthood and parenthood in the course of my interviews with younger and older men of various preliterate agricultural groups: the Lowland and Highland Maya, the Navajo, and the Druse of Israel and Syria. My purpose was to study the psychological features of later, postparental life; nevertheless, my male subjects spontaneously impressed on me the importance that parenthood had played in shaping their adult life and character. Routinely, my male informants would tell me that they had been wild in their youth: 'I didn't give a damn for myself or for anybody else. I was selfish, and thought only of my pleasure. [Clearly, you have changed much since then. What happened?] Oh, you know, I got married, I had kids'. Many of us have heard and even made the same banal and predictable statements. But cross-cultural repetition transforms a banality into a human universal and points to potent albeit extracultural – i.e., species – regulators of attitude and behavior. In this case, it points again to the universal importance that parents attach to the fact of their own parenthood.

I also found that parenthood sponsors standard comprehensions *about* parenting across cultures. Thus, while developmental psychologists may argue about the importance of early experience versus the 'here and now', illiterate peasants did not think it strange that, in my life-cycle interviews, I focused on such matters as weaning, toilet training, sibling rivalry, or the impact of a stepmother on character development. They already understood a great deal about the effects on the child's feelings, on the family's mood, and on the child's later development of these contingencies. When it comes to parenting, no human practice is inconceivably strange to any human group. My informants in a particular culture might disagree with me about the best child-rearing methods, but despite our ethnic, linguistic, and regional differences we *do* agree as to the range of possible child-rearing practices, from harsh physical discipline to *laissez-faire* permissiveness, and we generally agree as to the developmental consequences of these various styles. In sum, as a powerful standard experience – like love, or war – parenthood enforces its own universal norms and understandings, despite major disparities in cultural belief systems.

Gender Differences: The Parental Rationale

There also appear to be common understandings, cross-culturally, as to the distinctive roles of parental men and women. There seems to be general agreement that children need two kinds of nurturance, physical and emotional, that both these forms of security cannot – under average expectable human conditions– be supplied by the same provider, and that men should be largely responsible for the provision of physical security, while women should be largely responsible for the provision of emotional security. The evolutionary rationales for these sex distinctions are clear enough: women usually bear only one child at a time; but, to put it bluntly, one man can during the same time period inseminate many females. From the species or evolutionary perspective, men are redundant, hence more expendable than women. For this reason, and because of their larger muscles and greater natural endowment of murderous aggression, men are generally assigned to the high-risk, high-casualty tasks beyond the perimeter of the familiar, relatively secure community. To them fall the tasks of dealing with the world of strangers, beyond the confines of the domestic world, of being outwardly predatory, and of guarding against human and nonhuman predators. Women, being less expendable, are generally assigned to those settings in which they and their dependents are physically secure and in which they are freed to supply the experiences that foster the vital sense of emotional security, of basic trust, in their children.

This basic division of responsibility is recognized by most subsistence-level human groups. Thus, *Murdock's* [1935] tables, based on data from 224 subsistence societies, indicate that any activities requiring protracted absence from the home – be they hunting, trapping, deep-sea fishing, exploring, seafaring, or trading at a distance – are almost exclusively performed by men. Activities carried out in an intermediate zone, between the risky perimeter and the inner, domestic center (for example, dairy operations, erecting and dismantling shelters, harvesting, tending fowl) are in some cultures the province of men, in some the province of women, and in some societies they are performed by both sexes equally. However, activities carried out within the household itself, particularly those having to do with preparing and preserving food, are, regardless of culture, almost exclusively the responsibility of women. Clearly, it is not the capacity for hard labor that differentiates the sexes, but the *site* at which the labor is performed. Women often work much harder than men, but that work is by and large performed in settings where they can stay within reach and hail of their youngest child, settings whose security is guaranteed by the protective ring of men (even though these men may never be called on to fight).

But the standard requirements of parenthood not only organize the gender assignments of adulthood; they also organize and give content and meaning to the play, the education, and the socialization of boys and girls, long before their entry into actual parenting. Gender roles not only require particular behaviors; if these are to be predictable and trustworthy, then they must rest on a sound base of psychological structures and motives that are inculcated and quickened long before the actual behaviors are called for. Thus, *Barry* et al. [1957] have abstracted socialization data from ethnographic reports of 110 separate subsistent societies, and here again we find a striking transcultural consensus: Despite their cultural differences, these societies routinely recognize the female responsibility for children's emotional security and the male responsibility for physical security; and with striking unanimity they sponsor, through their socializing practices, the psychological traits that underwrite – when exercised in their proper domains – these forms of security. Thus, the central themes in female socialization are nurturance, responsibility, and to a lesser degree, obedience, while male children are almost universally (and exclusively) socialized towards achievement and self-reliance. In effect, girls are confirmed in the psychological counterparts and underpinnings of the mothering, emotionally-nurturing role, while boys are confirmed in the drive for achievement and exploit that will impel them beyond the safe confines of the home, the self-reliant qualities that will sustain them in their often risky and lonely forays beyond the perimeter.

Masculine attainment in these terms is generally tested in puberty rites, in *rites de passage*. As spectacles, these vary greatly in dramatic content and specific goals across cultures, but despite all differences they do seem to have a common aim: to test whether the boy has developed the psychological structures that are fundamental to the far-ranging life of the adult, parental male. In one form or another, the young candidate for manhood is subjected to an ordeal. If he endures it with some dignity, or at least without crying, then he has made it as a man, as a creature of the perimeter, and he is judged fit to join the adult males – whether as trader, hunter, sailor, soldier, rebel, itinerant worker, etc. – on some sector of the community's boundary. But if he shows weakness in the ordeal, if he in effect cries for his mother, then he has not accomplished the crucial transformation from child into man, from the life of the protected, domestic center, to the life ways of the perimeter.

Thus, members of each sex are trained to amplify, to transform into executive capacities, and to *enjoy* the emotional potentials that fit their gender assignments; and to discover, in the other sex, the qualities that are placed off limits for themselves. Men are shaped so as to relish their own capacity for rivalry, and to mistrust their conflicting tendencies toward empathy and sensuality, sentiments that could interfere with successful competition and achievement. But by the same token, they are allowed to relish and protect, in *women,* the very capacities that they have blunted within themselves. Likewise, women are urged toward being the center of harmonious social relations, and they come to distrust any competitive, aggressive potentials within themselves that are antagonistic to such important goals. Thus, younger women admire and *sponsor* male aggression (so long as it is directed away from themselves and their children), and they mainly live out their desires for exploit and competitive success through the spouse. (Thus men are urged toward war not only by the appetite for killing, but also by the quite realistic expectation that the women of their land will have sex with the soldiers of their land.)

Entering Parenthood: The Sharpening of Gender Distinctions
These gender divisions may remain relatively latent, even in the early, preparental years of marriage. Prior to parenthood, and despite their early and continuing training toward distinct sex roles, young men and women are allowed, in most societies, some freedom to indulge a wide and overlapping range of psychic potentials. Thus, prematernal women are often tomboys, while young men, including prepaternal husbands, can live out the extremes of their nature toward violence on the one hand and tenderness on the other. In effect, before parenthood young men and young women are allowed some freedom to live out their narcissistic strivings toward omnipotentiality – toward conserving, for the self, all possible potentials and options, no matter how mutually exclusive these might finally be. However, the entry into the condition properly called the 'chronic emergency of parenthood' leads to a mobilization in young parents of the structures that were laid down during early socialization, as well as a muting of the claims toward omnipotential satisfaction across all modes and zones.

Newton's [1973] formulations, based on cross-cultural data, help us to better understand the rationale for these crucial transformations. She has found that coitus, birth, and lactation – the three neurochemically regulated forms of female sexuality – while vital to successful reproduction and child rearing, are also tremendously vulnerable, likely to shut down in the face of outer threat. In order to proceed toward their reproductive goal these activities all require external buffering and protection, most often provided by men. In this vein, *Newton* cites ethnographic descriptions of young mothers in South America, the Middle East, and China, all pointing to a standard pattern of maternal engrossment with her infant, in an intense bond that can persist through the first few years of the child's life. At all these sites, the infant sleeps next to the mother and is nursed at the first sign of restlessness, and nursing takes precedence over any competing activity. Thus, it is not surprising that, across most societies, young men protect wives who are so engrossed in the reproductive act and so vulnerable because of it.

Ewing [1981], an anthropologist with psychoanalytic training, probed beyond the behavioral level, exploring the subjective side of Pakistani mothers' reactions to their own parenthood. She found that their investment in maternal behavior is matched by an internal repudiation of their aggression, which is seen as dangerous to their offspring: 'Young women chastise themselves for their own uncontrolled outbursts of anger. They are afraid of the harm their anger will cause their children'. The duty of the young mother is to submit to her mother-in-law, and to control any anger over this servitude for the sake of domestic harmony and for the sake of her children. However, her own passive defense against anger can go so far as to cause her to withdraw from contacts, even from those with her child. In this case the defense against dangerous anger, designed to protect the child, can have destructive consequences for that same child.

The predicted parental shifts are also noted for new American fathers. Thus, *Heath* [1972] found that first-time American fathers are significantly more hyperrational and vocational than their nonparental age peers. By the same token, they are *less* emotive and less affectionate than married non-fathers in the same age range. In other words, young men come to terms with their own parenthood by focusing on their role as provider, and by damping out the kinds of emotionalism that could interfere with that vital role. But these young men are not totally abandoning warm sentiment; rather, they are putting it on 'hold' and giving over the feeling function to their wives. In effect, they become more stereotypically *macho,* not in the service of male chauvinism, but in the service of their children's need for a reliable provider, one who will not be distracted by fluctuating sentiment from this stern and long-range purpose.

Studies of couples in first parenthood reveal similar findings. Thus, *Perloff and Lamb* [1980] found that, following the onset of parenthood, both partners in the marriage show increased sex-role stereotypy; and *Troll* [1977] found that, true to the same stereotypes, men do less housework after fatherhood than before.

An interesting if limited study was done under my direction by an Honors student at the University of Michigan. *Kupper* [1975] interviewed and gave projective tests to newly parenting and nonparental married student couples, and found again the predicted shift among the parental men toward disciplined careerism: Thus, their goals, no longer inflated by narcissistically grandiose expectations, were more realistic and more attainable than those set by their nonparental peers. Most interesting are the results from the projective test comparisons. Thus, the 'Heterosexual Conflict' card of the standard Thematic Apperception Test (TAT) battery was shown to both the parental and the nonparental groups, and the resulting thematic (by parental status) distributions demonstrated differences in the subjective management of male aggression, along predicted lines. The stimulus card depicts a young man partly turned away from a young woman who reaches toward him. While most informants see tension and discord in the scene, they vary in defining the sources of the couple's trouble. For the nonparental informants, the scene is one of domestic squabbling: The young man and young woman are not sharply differentiated by their personal qualities, nor by the intensity of their aggressive feelings toward each other. However, in the stories from the parental group, strong sex distinctions appear, particularly in regard to the location and management of aggression: their accounts feature extradomestic challenges – there is a war; there is a job that needs doing; some man has insulted the woman – and the aggressive response to these challenges is concentrated in the young man. His action is centrifugal: away from the woman, away from the domestic center, and toward the enemy or the opportunity that he glimpses on the periphery, beyond the actual card boundaries. For parents, aggression no longer exists as a tension between the couple, but has been dispatched, via the young man figure, to the outer world.

Conversely, any fearful concern over the young man's boldness is not found in him; instead, it is concentrated in the young woman figure, who tries to restrain the young man's reckless action. If he is all thrusting, phallic exuberance, then she is turned against such aggression, and shows concern for its potential victims. In other words, as predicted by our model, for the parental group the young man figure has become a creature of the perimeter, whose job it is to concentrate the dangerous intradomestic aggression of both partners, to export it away from the vulnerable household, and to discharge it beyond the periphery against human or inhuman enemies, or against the agencies of impersonal nature.

But if parental informants see the young man as moving out of the domestic zone, to station himself aggressively on the perimeter, then they also see women as moving back into the domestic precincts. Consider the responses to a card which shows, in a bucolic setting, a man who plows the soil, a pregnant woman who leans against a tree, and a young woman who stands in the foreground, half turned toward the farmer, and holding a book in her hand. Stories told by normal respondents to this card usually center on the actions and motives of the young woman: She is seen to be either moving away from the farm in pursuit of her own independence, or moving – usually motivated by guilt and filial responsibility – back toward the domestic center, to be with and to help her parents. In our sample, the nonparental informants were prone to see the young woman as ambitious and centrifugal, but the parental informants quite decisively placed her in the world of household and motherhood. Thus, young parents move male figures away from the household, and by the same token they remove women *from* the periphery, returning them to the very center of the domestic world.

Parenthood and the Transformations of Narcissism

Thus far, the admittedly spotty evidence does support our proposition concerning the centrality of parenthood as a prime mover of adult behaviors, attitudes, and personal adaptations. The parental effect is evident, in new parents, at all these levels of personal organization. Most importantly, parenthood brings about one of the most potent transformations of narcissism in the entire life cycle. It marks the point at which parents surrender a large piece of their own narcissistic claims to omnipotentiality and immortality and concede these to the child. All developmental advances represent a dialectic between *stasis* and *orthogenesis,* between continuity and change. In the parental transformation, continuity has to do with the fact that preparental goals, fantasies, and ambitions retain their previous priority; change has to do with the fact that these are in some important degree conceded to the child. In the parents' eyes, it is the child who has title to the treasure houses of the future and who should live forever. In effect, the entry into parenthood represents both the recognition and the acceptance of one's own life cycle and one's own mortality; the idea of one's own death is less shocking, less *obscene* than the idea that the child might predecease the parent. In sum, while we do not find a total reordering of the parental personality, we do propose that major changes take place, having to do with a reallocation of narcissism. The parents curb their own claims, having to do with their own gratifications, and instead devote themselves to meeting the full range of demands – for physical security, for emotional response, and for sensual pleasure – put to them by their idealized child. Viewed from the parental perspective, narcissism is not, as frequently supposed, a stubborn piece of our pathology; rather, it is a human relational mode that only reveals its true evolutionary and adaptive meanings when it is finally put, in its matured parental form, to the service of the helpless child.

The Postparental Man and Woman:
Standing Down from the Parental Emergency

The psychological changes that take place in response to the parental emergency are in sharp contrast to the typical personality changes that have been identified, for men and women, in later life. My own cross-cultural research [*Gutmann,* 1964, 1967, 1969, 1975] into the psychological parameters of the aging process, plus the investigations of ethnographers and sociologists into the more overt, social situations of the aged, all speak to a common finding: that the second half of life brings about a notable revision of the psychological postures – the ego-mastery positions – that characterize the earlier adult years. Thus, where younger men live an active mastery style thematic of disciplined competitiveness and productivity, older men gravitate to the passive and magical mastery states: they become more pacific, more oriented towards pleasurable consumption, and more diffuse in the cognitive sense. More specifically, where younger men see energy *within* themselves as a potential threat that needs to be contained, deployed toward productive aims, or to the service of the community's war-like purposes, older men see energy as existing outside of themselves, lodged in capricious secular or supernatural authorities. For younger men, power must be controlled internally and deployed externally *(Active Mastery);* but for older men, power must be manipulated and controlled in its external guise, so as to offset their own weakness *(Passive Mastery).* Finally, unlike the phallic younger men, the older men seek pleasure in the pregenital direction: They become particularly interested in food, pleasant sights and sounds, and undemanding human associations. Where younger men, guided by a calculus of profit and competitive advantage, look at the world instrumentally and rationally, older men take some incidental bonus of esthetic pleasure from their daily routines, and they indulge themselves by eliminating the boundary between wish and perception *(Magical Mastery).*

In short, just as the psychological endowment of younger men fits them for their excursions on the perimeter, the emergent psychological functions of older men fit them for a new, more domesticated life, at the communal center. They lose their combative edge and the capacity of seeking and coping quickly with stressful conditions that are adapted to the emergency demands of the perimeter; and they elaborate the more vegetative capacities, consummatory and affiliative, that are calibrated to the relatively predictable and secure conditions of the hearthside.

The shifts in male psychological positions, from an active to a more passive or autoplastic position, are charted in figure 1, which gives the age distribution of mastery styles for a variety of culture/TAT card combinations. This display requires a brief word concerning the analytic method, and concerning the TAT cards themselves (which were presented at all sites).

The *Rope Climber* card shows a muscular, possibly nude man who either climbs or descends a rope; the *Heterosexual Conflict* card depicts a young man and women in spirited though ambiguous interaction; and the *Desert Scene* presents an arid, unpeopled region, though showing some evidence of cultivation. Each card presumably poses an implicit question: regarding the subject's relation to male assertion and energy in the case of the Rope Climber card; regarding the nature of heterosexual relations and sex-role polarities in the case of the Heterosexual Conflict card; and regarding the subject's relation to an ungiving environment in the case of the Desert card. Each response was regarded as an implicit answer to the implicit card question, and was coded for the particular version of ego mastery, expressed through the story, in regard to such basic card issues. Thus, Active Mastery responses reflected a vigorous but realistic management of the basic card issue (the Rope Climber ascends the rope successfully, for a productive purpose, and in the face of competition); Passive Mastery responses reflected anxious, constricted, or avoidant handling of card issues (the Rope Climber is fleeing from a fire); and in Magical Mastery responses, core stimuli are misperceived so as to avoid confrontation with the basic card issues (the respondent turns the card on its side, and says that the Rope Climber is asleep).

Figure 1 shows the proportions of Active, Passive, and Magical responses for each age/culture group, as refracted by each card. It also shows that, across cultures and cards, younger men tend to have the highest proportion of Active Mastery responses, that these decline drastically in the older groups, and that they are replaced by Passive and/or Magical Mastery responses. These cohort differences are replicated, as intraindividual differences, in longitudinal TAT data from Druse and Navajo informants. Thus, even though societies vary among themselves as to the pacing and degree of

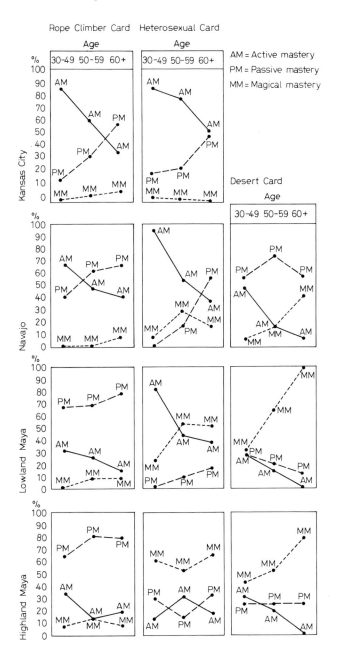

Fig. 1. Distribution of mastery styles by TAT card, culture, and age (reprinted from *Gutmann,* 1969].

change through the mastery styles the standard age sequence – Active, then Passive, then Magical Mastery – appears to be conserved for most societies.

The Virilized Postparental Woman

But perhaps the firmest finding in the study of aging personality concerns the psychological destiny of the older woman. Thus, whether in behavioral, projective, or ethnographic data, we find that women, across a wide range of cultures, age psychologically in a course opposite to that taken by men. Even in normally patriarchal societies, women become more openly aggressive in later life. Contrary to men, they become less interested in communion, less sentimental, more domineering, and more agentic. And just as the emergent passivity of men fits them for a new role, as brokers of *tabu* power, the heightened assertiveness of older women fits them for renewal as executives of their extended families. Continuing their investment in child-rearing, older women in effect graduate from primary care and into administration.

Thus, across time, across sex lines, and across societies, a massive postparental involution takes place: Reversing the pattern of the earlier, parental years (and consistent with the principles of Passive Mastery), the aging husband reenters – both physically and through his subjectivity – the domestic zone; and from his station there he becomes deferent towards those powerful figures, his wife as well as the gods, who command the wellheads of security. Through deference to his wife he guarantees his own security; and through ritualized humility he guarantees the spiritual security of his people. By these multiple changes, involving reciprocal developments in older spouses, there is ushered in the normal androgyny of later life.

Parenthood and Character in Later Life: A Tentative Model

Findings of the sort cited above are not new. Jung made the first clinical observations of what has been called the contrasexual shift of later life in the 1930s; and I, in collaboration with *Neugarten* in 1958 [*Neugarten and Gutmann*, 1968], was the first to study this effect empirically, in projective data from a normal United States population. I confirmed my American findings in cross-cultural studies in the 1960s and 1970s, and anthropologists who study the lifeways of elderly preliterates have also observed the contrasexual shift across a wide range of disparate societies. However, cultural anthropologists generally study one culture at a time; accordingly, they are prone to explain human behavior in externalized terms, as a reaction to social instigation at the local level [see *Brown,* 1984]. Thus, from the anthropological perspective, the role changes in men and women are given, in each case, a parochial explanation: they are seen as a response to particular cultural pressures or opportunities. But while anthropologists deal plausibly with the cultural particulars of later-life role change, they do not deal with the generic, transcultural phenomena – the virilization of the older woman, and the pacification of older man – that underlie and drive the particular behavioral changes in each case.

A model is required that would account for the distinct yet covarying trajectories of change across culture and gender. The conception of the parental imperative as the engine of personality change during the parental and postparental years accommodates available data – from men, from women, from a wide range of societies, and even from subhuman primates – in a parsimonious, unforced way. Thus, I have argued that the entry into parenthood mobilizes, for men and women alike, a readiness to value the child's needs over their own. In the service of the child's narcissism, parents give up the lingering illusion of personal omnipotentiality. They leave untended or turn over to their spouse those aspects of their own nature that would interfere with their particular role in parenting, and that would put their children at risk. Routinely, parents put their own capacities at the child's service until that time when the child demonstrates – usually by acquiring gainful work and/or a mate – that it can provide for its own physical and emotional security.

In effect, parents can relax when all of their own children are clearly on the way to becoming parental, or – as is often the case in peasant societies – when the oldest sons have taken over parental responsibilities toward the youngest, the dependent children still at home. At that point, as the sense of parental emergency phases out, parents can reclaim for themselves the narcissistic principle – the demand for omnipotentiality – that they temporarily abandoned in favor of their children, during the helpless years. They can assert the right – abandoned during the years of active parenting – to again know, live out, and experience all possibilities: agentic *and* communalistic; rational *and* sentimental; finally, masculine *and* feminine. Thus, during parenthood, men tended exclusively to their more instrumental, hyperrational, aggressive, and *masculine* side; but in the postparental period they claim the right to be feelingful, sentient, nutritive – in a word, feminine. By the same token, women claim title to the aggression that can no longer put their children emotionally or physically at risk, and that is less likely to drive away their now more dependent husbands.

In the postparental years adults finish paying their species dues: They no longer have to meet the psychological tax that is levied on our species in compensation for our children's freedom – their release from the programmed rigidities of instinct. Thus, the psychology of the later years may be marked not only by the sense of loss, but also by a subjective tension of liberation.

That is the general model, and in the final section of this chapter we will review research findings that support these propositions on the relationships between parental status and late-blooming features of personality. To this end, though a number of researchers [*Lowenthal* et al. 1975] have reported sex-role changes in the postparental years that conform to the predictions of our model, we will only consider in detail those which control for the contributions of aging per se, and thereby highlight the psychological effects, regardless of age, contributed by the postparental transition.

The Parental Model: Empirical Tests

The model outlined above predicts to more unabashed expressions of self-interest in the postparental years. Thus, *Galler* [1977] found that women returning in the middle years to professional life had always been achievement-oriented, but that their dormant ambitions had been quickened by the phasing out of active parenthood. She succinctly stated the essential issues: 'Women in the professional student group describe themselves as having kept their personal ambitions in the background for many years, supporting, instead, the career aspirations of spouses who are themselves professionals or academicians, as well as investing themselves in child rearing and adjunctive community activities. The "it's my turn now" attitudes verbalized by many of these returnees express a self-assertive rather than an other-directed attitude, an acceptance of their current limited interest in domesticity.'

Peskin and Livson [1981] conducted a particularly significant study, carefully sorting out psychological changes attributable to parenting stage per se as distinct from those attributable to chronological age. Inviting parental and older postparental adults to reminisce about their adolescent years, they then coded the resulting data for their thematic content. Their prediction, that current parental status would shape the recall of earlier experience, was borne out: Thus, regardless of age, actively parenting women tended to recapture memories clustered around nurturant and sentimental themes, while 'empty nest' women, again regardless of age, were more likely to stress memories that coded for power, dominance, and autonomy themes. Thus, the memories of actively parenting 40-year-old women resembled those of actively parenting 30-year-olds more than they did the memories of their postparental age-peers. A similar effect was observed for men: Actively parenting men remember their adolescent years as a time of competition and training for leadership, while postparental men from the same age cohort centered their adolescent memories around milder, more affiliative themes. Again, the memories of parentally involved 40-year-old men were more like memories of 30-year-old parents than like those of their postparental male age-peers from the same age cohort.

Peskin summed up the findings regarding older postparental women with the observation that the adolescent resources drawn on by this group are *'clearly for the self,* and not for the larger social unit' (italics mine). Similarly, healthy postparental men, by contrast to younger men (or older men who are still actively parenting), 'draw much more on affectively softer, generative, inward-seeking and cognitive dimensions'. Along similar lines, *Menaghan* [1975] found in a study of aging conducted among Chicago Irish, Italian, and Polish ethnic groups that childless men appear more passive, at any age, than men who are actively fathering.

Vatuk [1975] studied the Raya of the Rajput region of India. Again, stage counts more than age in demarcating the divisions of later life. Thus, women enter the age-grade of 'old age' – regardless of their actual years – when their children, and particularly their sons, get married. However, the Raya woman's transition into old age brings with it social gains rather than losses. Her son's marriage may 'age' her in the social sense, but it also brings her daughters-in-law who are pledged to her service; in particular, they do the 'inside' work, while the older woman now occupies herself with 'outside' work, on the interface between the family and the larger community. Vacating the woman's place in the domestic interior, the older woman can move, like men, to the social perimeter.

In sum, the foregoing studies, without explicitly testing it, do support the parental model: among other things, they suggest that older men may be kept 'young', in the psychological sense, by their continuing involvement, as fathers of young children, in the emergency phase of parenting.

Two recent studies by investigators other than myself have had as their avowed goal the testing of the 'Parental Imperative' model. Thus, *Ripley* [1984], in the course of her doctoral research, carried out a study of 60 Midwestern male industrial workers sorted into four groups: younger fathers, younger postfathers, older fathers and older postfathers (for both postpaternal groups the last child has been launched). These men were given projective tests and interviews from which an overall 'gender' score, ratings which reflected the degree of Active Mastery orientation, could be derived. In line with the Parental Imperative hypothesis, *Ripley* does find that gender scores reflecting an active, 'masculine' stance are highest for parental men, regardless of age, and lowest for the postparental men of either age group (a finding that is significant at the 0.005 level).[1]

Similarly, *Feldman* [1981] used the Bem Sex-Role Inventory to study fluctuations in the sexual orientations of Californian men and women across the stages of life from adolescence to grandparenthood. There are several problems with this study: it is based on cross-sectional data and is therefore very vulnerable to historical cohort effects (particularly given the large temporal range of subject ages, and given the culturally controversial nature of the variables, i.e., sex-role distinctions, under review). In addition, the BSRI, as a self-report questionnaire, does not tap the unconscious attitudes and motives that are perhaps most important in determining sexual orientation. As such, the BSRI could be particularly vulnerable to respondents' social desirability concerns – their wish to appear appropriate and particularly 'nonsexist' to liberal social scientists. Given these limitations, the authors' positive findings have to be read with caution:

> Gutmann's speculation that instrumental and expressive attributes are better understood as specific to stage of life rather than as traits affixed to one sex or the other receive some support from our data ... . The largest sex differences (on expressive factors) occur during the active parenting stages when in traditional families they serve to promote effective primary child care. The sexes describe themselves more similarly by the time that all their children have grown up and left home.

What is striking here is that the young parents, despite the massive pro-androgyny rhetoric that their generation has been subject to, nevertheless demonstrate the sex-role polarizations during the actively parenting years that are predictable from our model, the same changes that occur on schedule in more traditionally 'sexist' societies. In summary, however, because they are founded on projective tests and depth interviews, the results garnered by *Ripley* [1984] are more compelling than those reported by *Feldman* et al. [1981, p. 34].

[1] *Cooper* [pers. commun.], who is studying the TAT imagery of middle-class women, has developed preliminary findings, showing that postparental mothers tell much more vigorous stories than do parental women within the same age cohort.

The Druse Case: A Cross-Cultural Test of the Parental Model

Finally, my own field research among the Levantine Druse allows us to sort out with some strictness the effects of parental state versus the effects of chronological age in bringing about the characteristic male psychological changes of later life. As we have seen, in later life the focused, phallic organization of masculine personality tends to shut down in favor of a more diffuse spectrum of libidinal themes, including those that were salient in the earliest years of life. Thus, as figure 2 indicates, we find that the proportion of *pleasurable* references to eating (relative to all other oral material, including food production and preparation) in the individual interviews, when converted to a *syntonic orality* score (expressed as a percentage of the total orality score), shows much the same rate of increase with age ($p < 0.005$), across two very disparate societies, the Navajo (n = 87) and the Druse (n = 73). Thus, we can say that oral-incorporative interests, as estimated by the orality score, show much the same prominence in later life, across two very distinct cultures, that they presumably showed in early childhood.[2]

To test the possibility that parental status has an effect, independent of age, in determining the variations in passive dependency, we developed a quantitative scale to track the levels of parental involvement among Druse men, and we distributed the individual orality scores against the respondents' parental status. Figure 3 shows the distribution of orality scores by age and by stage of parenting, and indicates the powerful effect that male parenthood plays in determining the oral, passive toning of male Druse personality. Thus, for any age, men who are still actively parenting show lower mean orality scores than the postparental men ($p < 0.065$). While the level of orality remains relatively constant across age groups for those men who still maintain dependent children in their households, these same orality scores go up, dramatically, across all age groups, for the Druse 'empty nest' men. Again, it is not physical aging that brings on the psychological concomitants of aging; in this inner and more subjective sense, aging is in

---

[2] The orality score taps more than a sensory interest in groceries: it refers not only to the oral zone as a locus of pleasure, but also to the oral-receptive *mode* as a general feature of personality. Thus, we find that in later life other receptor sites begin to function as metaphors of the mouth: They become alternate centers for the passive intake of pleasant sensations. In effect then, the orality score indexes the generally passive-dependent tone of personality: for example, besides covarying positively with age, orality also correlates significantly with health ratings, and with active-passive ratings derived from the TAT stories and dreams of Navajo men.

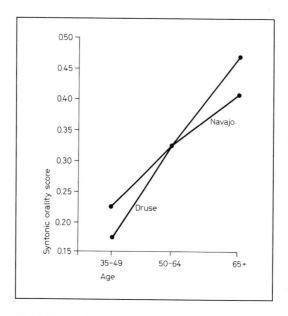

Fig. 2. Comparison of Navajo and Druse syntonic orality scores.

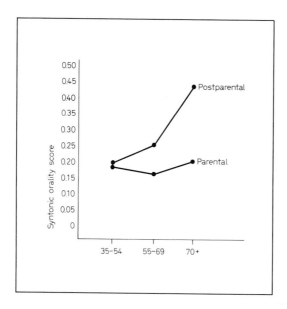

Fig. 3. Variations in syntonic orality by Druse parental status.

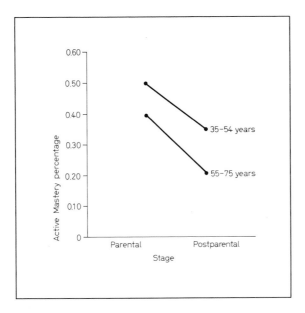

Fig. 4. Active Mastery by age and Druse parental stage.

some sense *chosen:* it comes about when men and women demobilize, or stand down from the parental emergency.

If we provisionally accept oral-incorporative tendencies as an index of narcissism, we can extend the meaning of these findings: they suggest a narcissistic recathexis of the self among postparental men who now wish to experience themselves (rather than their children or their dependents) as centers of pleasurable omniconsumption.

Similar results emerge when we consider age and parental status as independent variables, and distribute the TAT-derived ego mastery scores of 127 Druse males against these dimensions. These TAT scores quantify the proportions of Active, Passive, and Magical responses in the individual protocols, the hypothesis being that parental status would prove more powerful than chronological age in accounting for the variation in ego mastery scores. Specifically, we believed that the cessation of active parenthood (marked by the absence of dependent children in the respondent's household) would predict, more significantly than age per se, reduced scores on Active Mastery and elevated scores on Passive and Magical Mastery modalities. As figure 4 indicates, these expectations were, to a significant degree, borne out: analysis of variance reveals that actively parenting men are higher on Active Mastery than their postparental age-peers, while actively parental men in the 55 to 75 age range score higher on Active Mastery than postparental men in the age range 35 to 54. Though there are independent age and parental stage effects, the stage effects are more significant (age $F = 8.75$; stage $F = 18.38$, $p < 0.001$).

The predictions from the parental model are also borne out in regard to Passive and Magical Mastery, though there is an independent age effect registered in the sequencing of these mastery styles. Thus, figure 5 shows that younger (35+) postparental men move into Passive Mastery much more decisively than is the case with their older (55+) counterparts (the parental effect is significant at $p < 0.03$), while the opposite outcome holds in regard to Magical Mastery. As figure 6 illustrates, for that dimension, the mean scores of younger (35+) postparental men are actually *lower* than those of their actively parenting age-peers; but the mean Magical Mastery scores of the postparental older men (55+) are higher than those of any other cohort, including their still-parental age-mates (parental effect significant at $p < 0.06$).

In sum, most postparental Druse men, regardless of age, show reductions in Active Mastery; but younger postparental men move away from Active into Passive Mastery, while older postparental men, as they exit from Active Mastery, move directly into Magical Mastery, bypassing the intervening Passive Mastery stage. Again, the major thesis of the study is borne out, though in a somewhat qualified form: The postparental transition releases in men a renewed narcissistic demand for the kinds of sensory pleasures and diffuse cognitive modalities that they had muted in the service of their parental assignment; meanwhile, age, as an independent factor, determines the choice of postparental modalities – toward dependency and diffuse sensuality (Passive Mastery) for younger men, or toward egocentric forms of cognition (Magical Mastery) for older men. We can only propose a tentative explanation of the significant effect that age plays in determining the choice of postparental mastery styles. It may be that late fathers have always been invested in denial – particularly of their own aging – and that they maintain such denial in their middle years via protracted or 'off-time' parenting. In later life, facing an enforced retirement from parenthood, they may refuse the 'feminine' alternatives represented by Passive Mastery, and instead continue to maintain their denials in the more extreme form of Magical Mastery: that is, they misperceive the troubling realities that they can no longer avoid or deny through pragmatic activity.

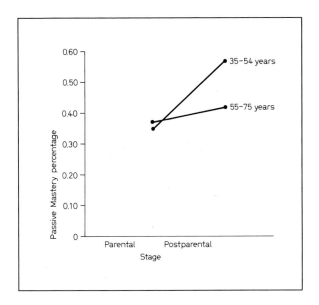

Fig. 5. Passive Mastery by age and Druse parental stage.

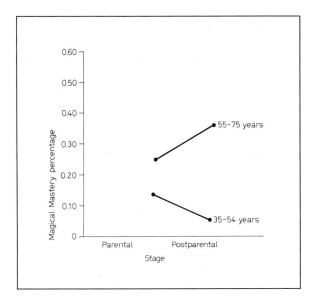

Fig. 6. Magical Mastery by age and Druse parental stage.

Parenthood and Aging Among the Primates

In sum, as we begin to test the Parental Imperative model across a variety of populations (including exotic cultures) we find that it is thus far supported without, to my knowledge, any disconfirming instance. Again, the parenting stage stands forth as a pivot of the adult sector of the life-cycle; and the psychological themes that attend parenting and its aftermath can be thought of in terms of their species/evolutionary as well as their purely personal significance. Thus, fluctuations in parental involvement across adulthood have standard consequences for inner affective states as well as outer role performance.

The centrality of the parental imperative is also borne out by recent observations of aging primates, particularly those undertaken by *Hrdy* [1981]. Such studies indicate that the sex-role consequences of the post-parental transition appear to be general, not only across the range of human cultures, but also across the range of primate species, nonhuman as well as human. Thus, some recent studies of aging among subhuman primates provide interspecies evidence for the clear developmental shift in the postparental female that was first identified through human, inter-cultural comparisons. Bear in mind that certain crucial similarities across the human and nonhuman primates allow us to make meaningful inter-species comparisons. Most significantly, all primates have in common the long dependency and vulnerability of infancy and childhood whose con-sequences for human parenthood we have already considered. For exam-ple, among the lower primates the infant has few motor skills, save for the capacity to cling to its mother's fur. Of necessity, then, adult primates – whether human or otherwise – have in common an intense parental orien-tation, and these concerns are particularly manifested in the behavior of reproductive females. Thus, like the majority of younger human mothers, the maternal ape in a variety of monkey species is devoted almost exclu-sively to the care of her latest, fur-clinging infant. She is at the same time relatively inoffensive in her dealings with other adults, mainly relying on dominant males, rather than on her own teeth and limbs for the physical protection of herself and her helpless infant. Thus, during the period of intense parenting, she allies herself with physically dominant males, and trades sexual access for their protection. However, in the postparental years, a striking change, reminiscent of our cross-cultural observations among humans, occurs among aging members of the most successful monkey species. *Hrdy,* who conducted field studies of the Langur and Macaque monkeys, noted that older monkeys support younger animals in ways which 'seem to vary with the sex of the animal and the situation of the group. Males generally bow out leaving older females to intervene actively in the fate of their descendants'. In effect, primate females enact both procreative roles: they provide physical as well as emotional security, though given the mutual exclusivity of these parts, they play them out sequentially, over the life cycle, rather than concurrently, within the same time frame. As *Hrdy* reported, 'When a troop of Langurs is threatened by dogs or humans, or by encroachments upon its territory by other Langurs, it is typically the adult males or the oldest females who leave the rest of the troop to charge and slap at the offenders'.

Clearly then, among certain species postreproductive primate females take up the defender's role that was supposedly reserved for young and vigorous males. The breeding mothers are almost exclusively providers of emotional security, but (like procreative adult males) the postreproductive female is a provider of both emotional and physical security. Having passed her procreative prime, she becomes, in the species sense, redundant and expendable; consequently, at times of danger she moves not to the protected center of the group, but outward, to join the male combatants on its defense line. There, older females take up the warrior's role that is off limits to the younger females. In sum, the older postparental females openly reveal the aggressive propensity that, earlier on, would have put their children at psychological risk, or threatened their mates. This aggressive power is vital to the older female's kin-tending role, and – in the human case – to their role as administrators of the extended families wherein the basic parental work is fostered.

Thus, when the primate female, human or nonhuman, exits from the active parental role, she does not end her significant life work, but instead begins a new and potentially more aggressive phase of existence, endowed with the psychological vitality that was much less available during the parental years (when she was physically more vigorous, but psychologically more inhibited).

In rough form, the fate of the older primate female illustrates the developmental design for older humans, both male and female: the ending of parental restraints releases unused, blunted potentials, and these are transformed by reciprocal psychosocial ecologies (the system of institutions, and mentors who recognize, require, and *recruit* the emergent potentials toward new roles) into new psychic structures: the executive capacities that serve self, society, and species in later life. In the next section we will consider this process, and its gender-related variations, in greater detail.

The Developmental Transformations of Late-Emerging Potentials

It is clear that the postparental growth potentials become more evident when we take a transsocial and even a transspecies sighting on later life, expanding our samples to include postreproductive primates, as well as postparental men and women. As one consequence of this review we now realize that the very term 'postparental' is inexact; given properly facilitating circumstances, older individuals become emeritus parents rather than ex-parents. They do not lose touch with the suprapersonal, species aspects of the life cycle; instead, the surgent potentials of later life bring about new connections with species goals, moving older people towards new roles, wherein they maintain the larger social and cultural ecologies of effective parenting.

This developmental view of aging does not rule out the dimension of loss. But many seeming losses of later life – much like those of earlier life – can be seen as the preconditions for further advance. Thus, men selectively lose the physical capacity and psychological appetite for taking life, and women lose the capacity and appetite for giving life; but as the psychophysiological systems that serve the emergency conditions of adulthood – e.g., war and childbearing – phase out, they reveal a previously hidden, vegetative physical and psychological organization. These changes uncover a body/mind format that is fitted to live in and to maintain *stable* social and physical environments. If younger individuals have bodies and motives that lead them to relish and provoke change, then older people have bodies and motives that lead them to relish and sponsor the equally vital dimensions of personal stability and continuity. Regarding men, *Griffin* [1984] finds that the change-provoking and stability-maintaining aspects of the social dialectic are partialled out among the generations; and by the same token, specific responsibilities in regard to the maintenance of social stability are portioned out among the sexes in later life.

In this regard, consider the generic roles of older women: as the cross-cultural and primate data make clear, older females move away from direct and primary infant care into administration – around the planet, wherever we find organized extended families, rooted in place and in history, then we will also find powerful matriarchs administering them, and insuring their continuity as centers of trust, of tradition, and of reliable parenting on the part of their component nuclear families. Moreover, the aggressive capacities released in postparental women are the necessary precondition for their expanded role as the eminence of the extended family. In sum, while the biological parents serve the immediate needs of their young children, the elderly matriarchs also play their vital part in the parental drama: parents as well as children must be sustained; and the extended family – as administered by matriarchs – provides a continuous support system for parents, and thereby insures the necessary decencies of that most demanding role. Precisely because she is now detached from active, hands-on parenting, the older woman can graduate to the next vital parenting level: the management of the extended rather than the nuclear family; and, by extension, of the individual parental couples within the extended family.

Just as older women maintain the vital aspect of family continuity via their kin-tending role, older men maintain the continuity of traditional and moral systems via their special role as culture-tenders. The seeming losses and regressions of the later years can, given facilitating circumstances, become the necessary preconditions for the developmental advances that are proper to that period, and that can only show themselves in full force at that time. To repeat, older men may lose the qualities of the warrior, but as these fade out they reveal an understructure of hitherto hidden cognitive and affectional potentials. 'Hardened' into fixed capacities, these are recruited to the service of self and society in the later years. Thus, as men give up the ways of the warrior, and their station on the community's perimeter, they move back towards the domestic world, there to rekindle qualities of sensuality, feelingfulness, and mildness repressed during their days of active fathering. Rather than restlessly seeking and provoking change on the perimeter, they seek constancy in terms of place, person, and nutriment at the protected center. However, in their minds they still reach out, beyond the familiar neighborhood to invest the supernaturals – the ultimate vessels of unwavering wisdom and nurture. Older men who have fallen back from the physical perimeter subsequently, as masters of ritual, move out to the spiritual perimeter, to confront the powerful and empowering gods. The strength that they no longer find within themselves, older men discover in the supernaturals; and they use prayer, a passive-dependent modality, to beseech, for themselves and for the people, their fire from the gods.

In the traditional setting, older men make the invisible but powerful presences that surround and penetrate the community real for themselves; and in so doing, they make them real for younger individuals who are otherwise too involved in pragmatic affairs to recognize or traffic with the gods. In effect then, older men draw back in order to advance: as they sink physically into the comforts and certainties of the center they at the same time move out in fantasy to invest and inhabit the spiritual frontiers of the community: the *tabu* gods, the traditions, and myths that reflect the people's history with their gods, and the rituals that connect the observing community to the gods.

In effect, even as they physically weaken, in the traditional community older men enter into the universal dialectic of power, which holds that death precedes rebirth, and that decrepitude is the precondition for strength. To inherit the strength of the gods, one must first – in token ways at least – be destroyed by them [*Gutmann* 1973]; and in the eyes of the traditional community the old man who has been wasted and weakened by the gods, becomes *as a consequence* a fit candidate for their *tabu* powers, and he is viewed by his community as a bridgehead to such power. He becomes the channel whereby the healing and fruitful powers of the gods are distributed into the community to refresh its vital systems.

Quite possibly, every viable society is founded on and draws its vitality and sense of uniqueness from a special myth, of special divine origins; and by linking the community to its sponsoring gods and their *tabu* powers, older traditional men recreate for others the climate of special mythic beginnings. They provide mythic connection, hence legitimacy, for the always unique system of shared, idealized understandings, permissions and constraints, that we know as 'culture'. Becoming culture-tenders, older men – like older women – support the parental institution of society, in a special, but most vital way. Where older women, via their assertiveness, manage the organizational contexts of parenting, older men, via the humility that ties them to the gods, manage the cultural systems which relate the pragmatic order to the mythic ideal, thereby providing the conformities and restrictions of daily social life with meaning and significance. When we recall that adequate parenting calls for great restraint, and for the surrender of omnipotential claims in favor of the child, then the relationships between culture, culture-tending, and parenthood become more clear. As *Erikson* once remarked, deprivation per se is not pathogenic; it is only deprivation *without meaning* that is psychologically destructive. By providing idealized meanings, a strong culture gives *significance* to the imposed deprivations that are the very essence of parenthood. Thus, to the degree that older men tend culture they too, like women, are still engaged in parenting: in them, the late life turn towards androgyny unmasks the latent skills and traits that fit them for special, gender-specific roles in the service of cultural stability and, by extension, adequate parenting. It is these maturations, rather than fortuitous adaptations to loss, that constitute the true developmental phenomena of later life.

Conclusion: Legitimizing the Field of Life-Span Human Development

Finally then, those studies which point to a 'parental' shaping of psychological processes in the later years, though far from complete, do suggest a productive direction for life-span developmental psychology, and a hopeful direction for geropsychology as a whole. To repeat, they provide refreshing alternatives to the catastrophic view of the aging process which holds that all later life changes, in men and women, are ultimately last-ditch adaptations to imposed loss and inevitable depletion. The 'Parental Imperative' hypothesis, by contrast, identifies the species-preserving as well as the individual-serving implications of late adult changes, and thus underscores their essentially developmental nature.

Most important, if new potentials are indeed released in later life according to some developmental design, then geropsychologists can begin thinking in new ways about services to the aged and their delivery. Instead of thinking about the aged as hapless recipients of services over which they can have little control, they can begin to study the ways in which postparental *potentials* can be transformed – into resources and capacities – not only for the elders, but for us all.

References

Barry, H.; Bacon, M.; Child, I.: A cross-cultural survey of some sex differences in socialization. J. abnorm. soc. Psychol. *55:* 372–432 (1957).

Ewing, K.P.: The crisis of marriage for two Pakistani women. Unpublished manuscript (Department of Anthropology, University of Chicago 1981).

Feldman, S.; Biringen, C.; Nash, S.: Fluctuations of sex-related self-attributions as a function of stage of family life cycle. Devl. Psychol. *17:* 24–35 (1981).

Galler, S.: Women graduate student returnees and their husbands: a study of the effects of the professional and academic graduate school experience on sex-role perceptions, marital relationships, and family concepts. Unpublished doctoral dissertation (School of Education, Northwestern University, Evanston 1977).

Griffin, B.: Age differences in preferences for continuity and change. Unpublished doctoral dissertation (Division of Psychology, Department of Psychiatry and Behavioral Sciences, Northwestern University Medical School, Chicago (1984).

Gutman, D.L.: An exploration of ego configurations in middle and later life; in Neugarten, Personality and later life (Atherton Press, New York 1964).

Gutmann, D.L.: Aging among the highland Maya: a comparative study. J. Pers. soc. Psychol. *7:* 28–35 (1967).

Gutmann, D.L.: The country of old men: Cultural studies in the psychology of later life (Institute of Gerontology, University of Michigan, Ann Arbor 1969).

Gutmann, D.L.: The subjective politics of power: the dilemma of post-superego man. Social Research *40:* 570–616 (1973).

Gutmann, D.L.: Parenthood: a key to the comparative psychology of the life cycle; in Datan, Ginsberg, Life-span developmental psychology: normative life crises (Academic Press, New York 1975).

Heath, D.H.: What meaning and effect does fatherhood have for the maturing of professional men? Merrill-Palmer Q. *24:* 265–287 (1972).

Hrdy, S.B.: 'Nepotists' and 'altruists': The behavior of old females among macaques and langur monkeys; in Amoss, Harrell, Other ways of growing old: anthropological perspectives (Stanford University Press, Stanford 1981).

Kupper, G.: Exploring the impact of parenthood on young college students. Unpublished Honors thesis (University of Michigan, Ann Arbor 1975).

Levy, R.I.: Notes on being adult in different places. Unpublished manuscript (Department of Anthropology, University of California, San Diego 1977).

Lowenthal, M.F.: Psycho-social variations across the adult life course: frontiers for research and policy. Gerontologist *15:* 301–307 (1975).

Lowenthal, M.F.; Thurner, M.; Chiriboga, D.: Four stages of life (Bass, San Francisco 1975).

Mandelbaum, D.: The world view of the Kota; in Marriott, Village India (University of Chicago Press, Chicago 1957).

Meneghan, E.G.: Parenthood and life satisfaction in later life: a comparative analysis. Unpublished paper (Committee on Human Development, University of Chicago, Chicago 1975).

Murdock, G.P.: Comparative data on division of labor by sex. Soc. Forces *15:* 551–553 (1935).

Neugarten, B.L.; Gutmann, D.L.: Age-sex roles and personality in middle age: a thematic apperception study; in Neugarten, Middle age and aging (University of Chicago Press, Chicago 1968).

Newton, N.: Psycho-social aspects of the mother/father/child unit. Meeting of the Swedish Nutrition Foundation, Uppsala 1973).

Perloff, R.; Lamb, M.: The development of gender roles: an integrative life-span perspective. Unpublished manuscript (Department of Psychology, University of Wisconsin, Madison 1980).

Peskin, H.; Livson, N.: Uses of the past in adult psychological health; in Eichorn, Mussen, Clausen, Hann, Honzik, Present and past in middle life. (Academic Press, New York 1981).

Ripley, D.: Parental status, sex roles, and gender mastery style in working-class fathers. Unpublished doctoral dissertation (Department of Psychology, Illinois Institute of Technology, Chicago 1984).

Vatuk, S.: The aging woman in India: self-perceptions and changing roles; in DeSouza, Women in contemporary India (Manohar, Delhi 1975).

Diversity and Function in Intergenerational Relations: A Symposium

Jeanne L. Thomas, Organizer

Contr. hum. Dev., vol. 14, pp. 62–64 (Karger, Basel 1985)

Introduction

Jeanne L. Thomas

University of Wisconsin-Parkside, Kenosha, Wisc., USA

Although one can adopt a life-span orientation in the study of any developmental process, this perspective is essential in the study of intergenerational relations. Consideration of mutual influences among age-related changes in different periods of the life cycle is inescapable; similarly, generational differences in cultural experience, and the developmental implications of these differences, are of primary interest.

Scholars from several disciplines have studied intergenerational relations. Issues addressed in earlier work include intergenerational proximity and frequency of contact, the content and affective quality of interactions, sources of conflict, intergenerational assistance patterns, and subcultural variation in intergenerational relations [for reviews, see *Bengtson and Cutler,* 1976; *Brubaker,* 1983; *Fogel* et al., 1981; *Sussman,* 1976]. The goal of this symposium was to discuss current work relevant to several of these issues, and to note emerging empirical and theoretical priorities. The symposium was first presented at the Annual Meeting of the Gerontological Society of America in San Francisco; *Gunhild Hagestad* of Pennsylvania State University kindly served as a discussant.

Presentation topics were diverse. *Bertram Cohler* discussed ethnic group differences in intergenerational relations, with special attention to the import of historical circumstances upon these bonds. *Dean Rodeheaver* described intergenerational support networks of the rural elderly, on the basis of an ethnographic study. Based upon exploratory research of grandparenting, *Nancy Datan* and I considered stability and change over time in intergenerational relationships. Finally, *Helen Kivnick* examined implications of intergenerational experiences for psychosocial growth.

Despite the variation in topics, there were recurring themes in findings and conclusions. One theme comprised descriptions of variation in intergenerational relations. All of the papers described temporal variation: in *Kivnick's* and in *Thomas and Datan's* papers change over time occurred primarily within the experience of members of one generation, while *Rodeheaver and Cohler* described variation related to more extended historical processes. Cultural variation was highlighted in two papers: *Cohler* noted the unique features of intergenerational relations in three ethnic groups, and *Rodeheaver* discussed intergenerational functioning characteristic of Appalachia. Finally, *Kivnick* emphasized the importance of attention to individual differences in investigations of intergenerational relations.

A second theme was that of functions served by intergenerational relationships. *Cohler, Rodeheaver,* and *Thomas and Datan* all described family assistance networks, noting both individuals' expectations about and reactions to intergenerational support. In *Kivnick's* work, emphasis was upon intergenerational bonds as contexts for reworking, preworking, and resolving psychosocial crises.

It is rarely possible for a published symposium to convey the dynamic qualities of the presentation session, when participants, audience, and discussants comment upon the papers. It is possible, however, to review the questions raised about individual papers. In considering these questions, at least one common theme is again apparent: the need for greater scope and depth in theoretical and empirical contexts for studies of intergenerational relations was implied.

Cohler's paper led to the question of differences in intergenerational relationship among emigrants from different regions within a single country (i.e., Northern vs. Southern Italy), a type of variation which was, according to *Cohler,* important in this area. As a discussant, *Hagestad* noted implications in the *Cohler* paper of subcultural differences in life course patterns, and thus in resolution of psychosocial issues. In considering the *Rodeheaver* paper, one wonders about the history of the support networks explored in the first study: as *Rodeheaver* noted, it is unfortunate that antecedents of the distinct assistance patterns were not examined in this study.

In response to the *Thomas and Datan* paper, the question of age differences in reactions to grandparenting arose. This question highlighted a basic feature of qualitative research: statistical analysis of the findings may be inappropriate, although such analyses could often enhance understanding of the issues raised in qualitative studies. A second question about this paper concerned bonds between great-grandparents and great-grandchildren, an area which the investigators had not had the opportunity to consider in the reported study. In considering *Kivnick's* work, *Hagestad* questioned the empirical implications: given the stress that *Kivnick* placed upon the individuality and uniqueness of grandparenting, how might appropriate research be designed?

Thus, the symposium provided an occasion for researchers and theorists of intergenerational relations to exchange perspectives. Consideration of this varied set of papers yielded two common themes – variations and functions – among findings and conclusions. Furthermore, at least one theme appeared among questions raised during the session: the need for broad and complex contexts from which the study of intergenerational relations is approached.

Contr. hum. Dev., vol. 14, pp. 65–79 (Karger, Basel 1985)

Aging in the Old and New World: Variations in the Peasant Tradition

Bertram J. Cohler

University of Chicago, Chicago, Ill., USA

Concern with the lives of older persons has dramatically increased across the past two decades. Much present discussion regarding both normative changes with aging, and also social policy designed to foster improved health and life satisfaction, has been based on findings regarding a particular generation or cohort of European-born older persons or the children of these European immigrants. Experiences in the Old and New World, including immigration and settlement in larger cities of the Eastern Seaboard and the Midwest of the United States, represent a dramatic change in social context from that of the Old World.

Changes in values, living standards, and modes of interpersonal relations, as a result of immigration and adjustment to a new society, all have affected the manner in which these persons have experienced aging. Differences in circumstances, time, and mode of immigration, together with differences in patterns of settlement in the New World, have further affected the experience of aging in the New World in ways which may not be as relevant for successive generations of better educated older Americans preserving ethnic ties in ways which are quite different either from the culture of the Old World or the ethnic traditions of first- and second-generation members of European ethnic groups.

Culture, Ethnicity, and Immigration

The concept of ethnicity refers both to intergroup relations between persons in a majority group and those in a minority, typically defined in terms of national origins [*Wirth*, 1928, 1945; *Handlin*, 1951, 1957; *Schmerhorn*, 1970], race [*Blalock*, 1967; *Van Den Berghe*, 1967], or religion [*Abramson*, 1973], as well as differences in value orientations or underlying cultural assumptions, leading to particular ways of perceiving and understanding experience [*C. Kluckhohn*, 1951; *LeVine*, 1973; *Cohen*, 1974]. When ethnicity is used to refer to intergroup relations, concern is generally with issues of social stratification, power, and authority. For example, *Yancey* et al. [1976] claim that urban residential patterns, in which persons of the same ethnic group live in proximity [*Lieberson*, 1963; *Heiss*, 1966], is a pseudophenomenon, arising as a consequence of residential segregation of minority group persons from higher status groups.

Explanations of ethnicity based solely upon intergroup relations neglect the powerful influence of culture, understood as the distinctive ways of life of a people [*C. Kluckhohn*, 1951], including preferred solutions for common existential dilemmas such as the relation among persons, the temporal focus of human life, or the relation of person and nature [*F. Kluckhohn and Strodtbeck,*1961; *Spiegel*, 1971]. While there is only a limited range of solutions to these problems available across cultures, preferred ordering of these solutions is distinctive for particular cultures. These distinctive solutions, together with associated beliefs and rituals, which organize personal and collective experience, providing meaning for life, become of particular significance at times such as immigration, when threats are posed to both the universality and adequacy of traditional modes for solving common existential dilemmas [*Wirth*, 1928; *Wallace*, 1956; *Kemper*, 1977].

As a consequence of increased contact with other cultures [*Smith*, 1960; *Barth*, 1969], particular solutions for basic human dilemmas, previously assumed to be universal, now become seen as particular variations which may not even represent solutions endorsed by a large number of persons. As a result of such cultural change, culture becomes aware of itself, leading to a sense of ethnic identity as a part of a collectivity of like-minded persons, as contrasted with others not sharing such views, and transmitted across generations within the family through socialization [*C. Kluckhohn*, 1959; *Weber*, 1968; *Spiegel*, 1971; *Devereux*, 1975; *Gleason*, 1980; *Hareven and Modell*, 1980]. Based on current formulations

[*Barth,* 1969; *Schmerhorn,* 1970; *Kolm,* 1971; *Greeley and McCready,* 1975; *Gordon,* 1978; *Petersen,* 1980], ethnicity may be defined as:

> Maintenance of particular customs and beliefs, based on particular solutions for enduring human dilemmas, transmitted through socialization across generations, leading to a sense of distinctiveness or 'peoplehood' in a society which is historically and geographically separate, and which are not necessarily continuous with contemporary traditions within particular societies of origin.

These enduring but evolving differences in preferred solutions for universal dilemmas foster differences across social groups which have been described as modal personality [*Inkeles and Levinson,* 1954; *Inkeles,* 1961] or ethnic personality [*Devereux,* 1975]. Even after several generations of residence in the United States, persons descended from particular European nations still identify with that heritage [US Bureau of the Census, 1971, 1973, 1983; *Greeley,* 1971, 1974; *Abramson,* 1973].

Two other aspects of this definition of ethnicity should also be noted. In the first place, particular cultural traditions are altered as a consequence of immigration. Later historical events within the new land lead to further shifts in these folkways. For example, *Hansen* [1952] has described a phenomenon among the third-generation members of Scandinavian ethnic groups in which there is a striking return to the traditions of the first generation. Consistent with *Wallace's* [1956] emphasis upon older traditions as a means of protection against 'mazeway disintegration', or loss of capacity to resolve problems in the face of social change, persons may rely on older traditions which, in past times, provided security when confronted with challenge. The current popularity of oral history and preservation of older craft traditions, reflected in the popularity of the Foxfire volumes on Appalachian life, may be an indication of the revitalization of older traditions at a time of rapid change in American society.

In the second place, there may be significant variations within particular ethnic groups both as a result of particular patterns of immigration, back-immigration, and return to the United States over time, and also as a result of increasing intermarriage with members of other ethnic groups across generations [*Kennedy,* 1944, 1952; *Baron,* 1946; *Greeley,* 1974; *Alba,* 1976, 1981], as well as increased secondary group activities such as participation in voluntary association and involvement in the workplace. To date, there has been little study of variations in beliefs or social relations across successive cohorts from particular sending societies.

The European Peasant and the New World

Over the course of more than 350 years, from the first colonies at Jamestown and Plymouth Plantation until the past two decades, the history of immigration to the United States has been that of the European peasant. Historically, 65–70% of all immigrants to the United States have come from rural Europe [*Rubin*, 1966; US Bureau of the Census, 1973].

Readable accounts of the history of European immigration to the United States have been provided by *Hansen* [1940], *Handlin* [1951, 1957], and *Olson* [1979], while discussions of particular ethnic groups are included in *Thernstrom's* [1980] encyclopedic volume. Most discussions of this European immigration distinguish between the colonial period, the early 19th century, and two later periods of active immigration – the 'old immigration' between the years 1830 and the Civil War, and the 'new immigration' across the last two decades of the 19th century – until the First World War. Indeed, only since 1945 has the ratio of European to non-European immigrants shifted in favor of persons from the Pacific and the Western Hemisphere.

The so-called old and new immigrations correspond to quite different traditions in European society termed by *Schooler* [1976] 'the legacy of serfdom'. As a consequence of serfdom, the serf or small farmer was bound to a lord, and to the larger hierarchical social order of which the lord was a part, through a complex set of obligations and restraints which resulted in complete subjugation of serf to lord together with lack of individual initiative and autonomy [*LeGoff,* 1980]. Serfs were expected to till and plow in common, as required both by custom and the agricultural practices of particular lords. As a result of this social organization of peasant life, serfs were provided with little opportunity for participation in decision making, leading a routine existence characterized by lack of personal initiative and self-direction, which fostered cognitive rigidity [*Schooler,* 1976].

Across Europe there was marked variation in the extent to which feudal social organization was adopted, as well as in the duration over time of this form of social organization, from Scandinavia, where feudal traditions were never established, to England and Ireland, where serfdom was abolished in the early 17th century, during the reign of James I, to Poland, Russia, and the Eastern states of the German empire, where serfdom was gradually abolished across the first half of the 19th century, and finally to Italy, south of the Po River, where serfdom was only abolished after Italy's inclusion in the Austro-Hungarian empire. Serfdom appears to have continued in practice until well after the end of the Second World War [*Banfield,* 1958; *Galtung,* 1971].

Consistent with this social psychological perspective on the legacy of serfdom, *Schooler* [1976] has shown that persons from European ethnic groups in the United States marked by an earlier end of serfdom also show more more effective intellectual functioning, increased cognitive flexibility, greater self-direction and emphasis of self rather than others as the origin of actions, increased emphasis upon intrinsic rather than extrinsic work styles, endorsement of less authoritarian and ethnocentric social attitudes, and increased sense of moral commitment. These differences appear even when controlling for social status but are associated with Catholicism. Significantly, the legacy of serfdom is also associated with time of immigration to the United States: it is particularly characteristic of the new immigration, especially across Southern and Eastern European Catholic groups, while it is largely absent both in the colonial tradition as well as in the old immigration of Scandinavian and Irish-Catholic groups.

This continuum of the tradition of serfdom, as presented by the old and new immigrations across the 19th and 20th centuries until the First World War, provides a useful means for understanding the formation of ethnic groups in the United States as sociohistorical events. For the present discussion, three European ethnic groups, the Irish-Americans, the Italian-Americans, and the Polish-Americans, have been singled out for particular study. Since all three are Catholic groups, it is possible to consider immigration and adjustment to the New World separate from differences imposed by religious background. Further, these three ethnic groups represent the process of immigration during the 19th and early 20th centuries and also show varying degrees of immersion in the legacy of serfdom: the Irish-American group is characterized by membership in the old immigration and did not significantly participate in the legacy of serfdom, while Polish- and Italian-American ethnic groups belong to the new immigration and participated more directly in feudal social organization. Indeed, the Italian-American group comes directly from this tradition while, for the Polish-American group, serfdom had ended a century prior to immigration.

The impact of the colonial tradition in the United States has been markedly disproportionate to the actual number of immigrants involved. From the first seaboard settlements until the beginning of the old immigration after 1830, there were only about 1 million English and Scotch-Irish settlers [*Easterlin,* 1980]. The realization of English politics and culture, expressed in the Protestant Ethic [*Weber*, 1958], of which Ben Franklin was the ideal type, emphasized worldly success both as a demonstration of the likelihood of being one of the elect and also as a means of showing the glory of god through 'this worldly asceticism' rather than 'other worldly asceticism'. Rational, methodical planning and emphasis upon future attainment was believed to be necessary in order to provide the most certain basis for future success [*Spiegel*, 1971; *Waterman*, 1981].

Aging and the Peasant Family in the Old and New World

Findings from observational and systematic studies have shown that differences in solutions for basic human problems continue in American society [*Etzioni*, 1959; *Gordon*, 1964, 1978; *Suttles*, 1968; *LeVine and Campbell*, 1972]. However, these differences are not constant over time. Just as changes may be observed between the preferred order for solutions to universal dilemmas when contrasting the historic value orientations of particular sending nations with those of European ethnic groups in America [*Spiegel*, 1971], there have also been changes in these solutions within particular ethnic groups in American society across generations or cohorts [*Hansen*, 1952; *Gans*, 1962; *Cohler and Grunebaum*, 1981]. Transmission of these value orientations, which provide the basis for cultural pluralism in American life, is largely a function of preadult and adult socialization within the family [*Mindel and Habenstein*, 1976; *Hareven and Modell*, 1980; *Cohler and Grunebaum*, 1981].

Immigration, which transforms culture into ethnicity, also leads to changes in social organization within the family which are discontinuous between the Old and New World [*Spiegel*, 1971; *Vecoli*, 1972; *Woehrer*, 1982]. Particularly among the Irish and Italian ethnic groups, the position of older parents within the family has shown dramatic reversals from the Old to the New World.[1] Among Irish farm families of the West counties, although social security has lowered the retirement age [*Streib*, 1972], it is not uncommon for those offspring selected to run the family farm to be in

---

[1] Interesting comparative findings have been provided in *Palmore's* [1980] compilation on the contemporary status of the aged in European societies, including reports by *Fleetwood* [1980] on rural and urban Irish aged, *Florea* [1980] on the continuing problems imposed on older Italians unable to continue working to support the family, and *Dobrowski* [1980] on aging in a communist society. These reports also show the dramatic strains on health and social services imposed by a rapidly aging society.

their mid-forties and still single, when the older parental couple retires from active management [*Arensberg and Kimball,* 1968]. From the early 19th century, the possibility that offspring could emigrate relieved pressure on the older parental couple to relinquish control [*Streib,* 1972].

Among Irish families in the United States, little of this traditional power of the parental generation may be observed; rapid social mobility [*Greeley,* 1972, 1974] and changes in help provided among urban families [*Biddle,* 1976] led to dramatic changes in the role of the older family member in Ireland and the United States. Stated in terms of *Kluckhohn and Strodtbeck's* [1961] and *Spiegel's* [1971] discussion of variations in value orientations, the first-ranked preferred solution for relations among family members in the Irish family shifted from lineal in the Old World to individualistic in the New World, leading to reduced power exercised by the older parents.

Even more dramatic changes, leading to enhanced rather than reduced status for older persons, may be observed within the Italian family in the Old and New World. In contrast with Irish farm families, Italian peasants neither owned nor lived on their land. Rather, they lived along with other families in dense settlements known as agro-towns [*Boissevain,* 1966] and worked on rented plots often widely scattered in the district. Abject poverty across many generations enhanced suspiciousness of others, leading to what *Banfield* [1958] characterized as amoral familism, maximizing the gains of the nuclear family at the cost of ties to kindred. Older family members, less able to contribute to the household economy, were regarded as a burden. Further, there was danger that these older parents might inform siblings and other kindred regarding any good fortune, leading to demands for sharing and assistance which could soon deplete family resources. Similar impact of poverty upon family relations has been described in *Stack's* [1974] ethnographic study of Black welfare families in the United States.

Clustered settlements led to particularly rapid communication, and as first villagers emigrated they sent back word of the opportunity in the New World, providing first-person testimony when returning for relatives. These first settlers from the agro-town provided a ready access to housing and jobs, fostering a process of chain migration [*McDonald,* 1956; *McDonald and McDonald,* 1964]. Already familiar with urban life, Italian families immigrated to the larger cities of the Eastern Seaboard and Midwest [*Ward,* 1971; *Golab,* 1973; *Verbaro,* 1973]. Often, several generations of relatives from the same family and village lived together in an apartment building, sharing resources and assistance in ways which were quite different from those of the Old World [*Gans, 1962; Ziegler, 1977; Cohler and Grunebaum,* 1981].[2]

Living in an industrial society, older persons could still make a contribution, both through participation in factory work and in caring for children and household so that younger family members could be free to work. The preferred solution for relations among family members changed from the more individualistic solution characteristic of Southern Italy to a collateral organization in the United States in which older family members were able to make significant contributions to the quality of family life, including transmission of beliefs and practices so important in the preservation of traditions of the Old World customs in the United States [*Gans, 1962; Bianco, 1974*].

While immigration resulted in the dissolution of the traditional extended Irish farm family and the emergence of a modified extended family from among the Italian-American family [*Litwak, 1965*], immigration had much less impact upon social organization of the Polish family in the Old and New World. In ways similar to the Irish peasant family, the Polish peasant lived on a family farm rather than in urban settlements. However, language differences and differences in customs, including the long tradition of serfdom, meant that immigration to the New World was much more difficult for the Polish peasant than Irish peasant.

Over time, the Church Parish emerged as a particularly salient force in immigration [*Thomas and Znaniecki, 1918–20; Lopata, 1976; Kantowicz, 1975*]. Reliance upon corporate decisions on the part of the Parish, including the first decision to emigrate, led over time to reliance upon the Church and other civic organizations as the major sources of support for new immi-

---

[2] While some critics of urban life [*Lieberson, 1963; Heiss, 1966; Yancey* et al., 1976] have argued that inner city ethnic communities were merely a result of residential segregation, perspectives based on social stratification fail to consider the significance for personal adjustment from continuing face-to-face relations with others sharing common values and folkways. The importance of such neighborhoods is demonstrated in *Gans's* [1962] and *Fried's* [1973] reports of the lives of Italian-Americans uprooted from Boston's West End as a result of urban redevelopment. *Suttles* [1968] has documented the extent to which urban redevelopment in Chicago has affected a variety of ethnic groups. Among the most serious effects of such urban change is the disruption of long-standing family ties. Although not necessarily characteristic of relations between the generations in Europe, processes of chain migration and processes of settlement in ethnic ghettos [*Wirth, 1945*] had intensified family ties characterized by interdependence, which contrasted with characteristic American emphasis upon individuality and personal achievement [*Clark, 1972; Waterman, 1981; Cohler, 1983*].

grants. Well-functioning voluntary associations, tied to the Church, buffered members of the Polish community from many of the problems of the larger society [*Sandberg, 1974; Lopata, 1976; Wrobel, 1979*].

The position of the older Polish family member was little changed between the Old and New world. In a society in which all available land and possessions had long since been distributed, redistribution and accumulation of additional possessions could only be realized through marriage, emphasizing the importance placed upon collateral relations as the preferred solution for the dilemma of human relationships in the Old World, a solution which has been maintained within the New World. In both the Old and New World, name and good reputation of older family members, as well as material goods accumulated over a lifetime by older family members, have provided an important source of status for younger family members. Since so much of cultural transmission takes place through the Parish, the role of older family members as a source of information regarding customs is less important within Polish than within Italian families, where traditional suspicion of the Church reinforced by traditional Irish-American control of the Church has been maintained in the New World.

Ethnicity, Personality, and Aging

While there has long been interest in so-called national character [*Kardiner, 1945; Benedict, 1946; Gorer and Rickman, 1950*] or modal personality [*Inkeles and Levinson, 1954*], findings reported by *Greeley and McCready* [1975] provide little support for assumptions regarding personality differences associated with particular ethnic groups based on European backgrounds. Differences between these ethnic groups and their traditional homelands, as well as among generations in the United States, appear to be more important than modal personality characteristics of country of origin. Even when research has shown some consistent differences in personality among ethnic groups, as in comparative studies of Irish and Italian Americans [*Opler and Singer, 1956; Opler, 1959; Zborowski, 1969; Stein, 1971; Cohler and Lieberman, 1977/78*], little of this research has focused on personality changes across different points in the life course or on contrasting generations or cohorts of persons from within particular ethnic groups.

For example, as in most aspects of the study of aging and ethnicity, most studies of personality and aging among particular groups have been based on cohorts of older persons with little formal education, often born in the Old World and suffering from the inevitable conflict in values between the Old and New Worlds [*Wallace, 1956; Chance, 1965; Cohler and Lieberman, 1977/78*]. *Mostwin* [1979] notes that older Polish respondents are particularly concerned that remembered traditions from the Old World be continued, especially fluency in Polish and perpetuation of the everyday services of the traditional Polish Parish Church.

Preservation of holiday rituals appears less salient in fostering morale on a day-to-day basis, for these older immigrants, than might be expected. *Clark* [pers. commun., 1971] notes that older Japanese- and Mexican-Americans are also less conversant with ritual objects and occasions from their homelands than might be expected. *Mostwin* [1979] reports that morale among older (immigrant generation) ethnic respondents was largely determined by age and quality of leisure after retirement. *Cohler and Lieberman* [1977/1978], comparing older persons with Irish, Italian, and Polish ethnic groups (and considering effects due to generation of residence in the United States), report that all three first-generation ethnic groups, regardless of immersion in the legacy of serfdom in the homeland, maintain a suspicious stance towards the world, relying on defenses of externalization and projection in dealing with inner conflicts. Further, Irish first-generation respondents report greater life satisfaction and fewer psychological symptoms than members of the two other ethnic groups, although membership in the Irish group is also associated with greater income and higher educational attainment, making it difficult to determine the extent to which these social background factors contribute to findings regarding life satisfaction.

Across Polish and Irish second-generation ethnic groups, particularly intense concern is expressed regarding attainment of satisfying personal relationships and in realizing successful achievement in the larger world. Older second-generation Italian-Americans continue to express the suspiciousness noted by several students of personality and ethnicity as a modal trait for this ethnic group [*Greeley and McCready, 1975*]. In a later report studying the midlife transformation to increased interiority [*Neugarten, 1973, 1979*], a process marked by increasing concern with the inner world and increased egocentricity as a consequence of a foreshortened sense of time [*Munnichs, 1966; Marshall, 1975; Gutmann, 1975, 1977*] among middle-aged men and women from these three ethnic groups, *Cohler and Lieberman* [1977/78] report that older first-generation Irish men show less change in the direction of an expected increase with an interior and passive orientation to the world than men from the Italian and Polish groups.

Aging, Ethnicity, and Delivery of Services to Older Persons

To much the same extent that present understandings of ethnicity in the United States have been based on the European experience, much of what is believed to be significant regarding psychological changes taking place with aging, including problems in obtaining health and social services, have been based on study of a cohort of older foreign-born persons with little formal education and, as a result of early socialization in the legacy of serfdom, problems both in being able to obtain and accept assistance.

As a last generation of older persons born in the Old World or children of parents participating in the Great European March is diminished through death, an era will end in which largely European-born elderly had required particular assistance in the use of health and social services. Figures from the 1970 census show that about a third of all foreign-born persons in the United States were over age 65 and comprised about 15% of all persons over age 65; by 1975, only 25% of all foreign-born persons were over age 65, comprising 12% of all foreign-born persons, while *Gelfand* [1982] estimates that, by the end of the 1980s, the proportion of older persons who are foreign both will drop to less than 5%. In 1970, an additional 16% of persons over age 65 were second-generation residents in the United States.

To date, much of what is known about psychological changes with aging, including findings regarding cognitive functions, showing increased rigidity with age, and social attitudes, showing increased conservatism and ethnocentrism with age, has been based on the generation of older persons from the new immigration, primarily those from the legacy of serfdom, leading to particular problems in distinguishing between cohort and aging [*Chown*, 1961, 1968; *Botwinick*, 1977; *Neugarten*, 1977; *Palmore*, 1978; *Baltes* et al., 1979]. It is to be expected that older persons socialized from earliest childhood into the world view characterized by the legacy of serfdom would continue to express the ethnocentrism, discomfort with ambiguity, and difficulty in solving complex problems which characterize both the legacy of serfdom [*Schooler*, 1976] and personality and cognitive changes associated with aging.

To date, there has been little systematic documentation of changes in the use of health and social services across generations of European-born older persons and their aging children and grandchildren. It has been assumed that rapid social change such as results from immigration and consequent 'mazeway distortion' [*Wallace*, 1956] may be associated with impaired mental health, increased psychophysiological symptoms, and lowered morale, leading to increased use of health and social services. Previous findings have suggested that the experience of immigration is both particularly stressful and is associated with lowered morale and increased psychiatric symptoms (and that these symptoms are a function of immigration rather than of preselection of otherwise less well adjusted persons) [*Odegaard*, 1932; *Murphy*, 1965, 1978; *Malzberg*, 1968; *Cohler and Lieberman*, 1977/78].

Findings reported by *Bengtson* et al. [1975] suggest that older persons may be particularly affected by social change, since modernization inevitably is accompanied by devaluation of older persons. Such generalizations may be less useful when, as a result of social change such as immigration, the status of older persons is increased rather than decreased. Further, as *Hansen* [1952] and *Wallace* [1956] have suggested, one effect of social change may be a revitalization movement in which there is increased emphasis upon values understood by an ethnic group as traditions. Revitalization movements enhance the status of older persons who become repositories of tradition regarding beliefs and rituals. At least in part, the social conflict experienced by immigrant groups in the United States, leading to increased reliance upon remembered traditions of the Old World as a means of coping with such conflict, has enhanced the status of older family members.

Across generations, continued emphasis upon the old ways has been important in buffering the effects of life strain as members of European ethnic groups have moved out beyond older neighborhoods, becoming part of the larger society. It may be for this reason that the third generation shows increased involvement in religion, as noted across a number of studies [*Hansen*, 1938, 1952; *Greeley*, 1972, 1974; *Gelfand and Fandetti*, 1980]. Survey findings reported by *Fandetti and Gelfand* [1976], concerning urban-dwelling Italian- and Polish-American ethnic groups, show that Italian-Americans, particularly those within the third generation, were more likely than Polish-Americans to believe in the importance of the family as the primary source of care and support for older persons. Further, reflecting differences in the use of both voluntary associations and formal organizations within Italian and Polish ethnic groups, due to differences in Old World culture as well as particular patterns of immigration to the United States, Italian-Americans have traditionally been doubtful that the Church or other institutions could provide care for older persons equal to that provided by the family. Similar findings have been reported

both by *Krause* [1978] and by *Cohler and Grunebaum* [1981] on the basis
of detailed interview and observational studies of Italian-American families.

Contrasting second-generation Italian-Americans choosing to live in
the suburbs or remaining in the traditional urban neighborhoods, *Gelfand
and Fandetti* [1980] report that suburban ethnic residents are much less
willing to have older persons live in their households, and tend to rely on
the Church as a source of assistance to a greater extent than among urban-
living second-generation Italian-Americans. Limitation in the ability of
both husband and wife to work outside the home is cited as a major problem resulting from having older parents living in the same household. To
date, little is known about personal and social characteristics of persons
choosing to move to the suburbs as contrasted with those choosing to continue living in urban neighborhoods or of possible changes over time in the
attitudes of suburban and urban second-generation Italian-Americans.

Findings first reported by *Thomas and Znaniecki* [1918–1920] and
more recently by *Sandberg* [1974], *Kantowicz* [1975], and *Lopata* [1976]
suggest that Polish-Americans have relied upon political institutions to a far
greater extent than Italian-Americans in solving problems, including care of
older persons. Ironically, although the extended family was of greater significance in the daily life of the Polish peasant than of the Italian peasant,
with immigration to the United States Italian-Americans developed a modified extended family [*Litwak*, 1965], available as a resource for older persons, while Polish-Americans increasingly relied upon community rather
than family as a source of support and assistance.

Older Italian-American family members are particularly likely to be
expected to provide assistance for a large social network of relatives and
friends, many of whom come from families who lived together in the same
village in the Old World, emigrating to the United States through chain
migration. Suspicion of civic and formal organizations (reflecting continuity in at least one respect between traditional Italian society and the Italian-
American ethnic group, particularly striking when contrasted with the
reliance upon extrafamilial institutions within the Polish-American community) further increases the expectations by family and friends for help
and assistance by older family members within the Italian-American ethnic
group. The degree of interdependence expected from these older Italian-
American family members may seriously tax available time and energy
[*Femminella and Quadagno*, 1976; *Krause*, 1978; *Cohler and Lieberman*,
1977/78; *Cohler and Grunebaum*, 1981].

Reliance upon family rather than institutions beyond the family as a major source of support and assistance across the life course has costs as well as benefits. Studies of older persons [*Rosow*, 1967, 1976; *Wood and Robertson*, 1976; *Cohler*, 1983; *Cohler and Lieberman*, 1977/78; *Cohler and Grunebaum*, 1981] have noted the extent to which older persons experience expectations for support and assistance as burdensome and intrusive, diverting time and energy from other areas of life which are important for these older family members. Findings reviewed by *Lowenthal* [1964] and *Lowenthal and Robinson* [1976] suggest that older persons experience their own lives as much less socially isolated than as viewed by younger persons. Older family members may not necessarily enjoy contact when arranged without sufficient regard for their own needs and plans.

While in general, as *Uhlenhuth and Paykel* [1971] have shown, the number of reported stressful life events may decline with age, such findings fail to include differing extent of immersion, across ethnic groups, in a network of family and friends portrayed by *Plath* [1980] as consociates. As *Cohler* [1983] and *Pruchno* et al. [1984] have shown, the greater involvement in a network of such consociates, the greater the number of demands for assistance and support experienced by older persons and the greater the exposure to eruptive and hazardous or stressful life events among consociates, such as financial reversals, illness, and deaths. Demands upon the time of older persons may be so great that marked strain is experienced as a result of attempting to meet the competing demands of parent, spouse, and confidant; such strains may contribute to the lower level of morale reported within the group of older Italian respondents as contrasted with the Polish and Irish ethnic groups [*Cohler and Lieberman*, 1977/78]. This description of older persons, particularly within the Italian ethnic group, as still very actively engaged in caring for others is in marked contrast with the stereotype of the older person in American society as only the recipient, and not the provider, of assistance to the child and grandchild generation.

Conclusion

Social psychological study of older persons from European ethnic groups raises fundamental questions regarding both the significance of ethnicity in American society as well as of the problems in differentiating the effects of cohort and age in understanding personality and intellectual changes across the second half of life. Until the past two decades, the majority of immigrants to the United States have been from European countries and, particularly across the past half century, countries in which the legacy of serfdom was most entrenched. This mode of social organization, emphasizing passive compliance to authority and lack of decision making in a highly stratified society, has had important implications not only for the manner in which these immigrants have become involved in American life but also for a particularly ethnocentric and inflexible stance towards interpersonal relationships observed as these immigrants aged.

The present generation of older persons identified with particular ethnic groups, better educated than counterparts in former times, is likely to differ from these historically earlier cohorts not just in terms of modal personality characteristics but also in terms of expectations of social services and use of health facilities. Some characteristics associated with outlook on life and particular value orientations do appear to have been maintained over time. While Italian-Americans have continued to rely on extended family ties as a major social resource in dealing with urban life, Polish-Americans continue to be more likely to rely on more formal institutions such as the Church. While particular traditions may have changed over generations of immigrants and their descendants, a sense of ethnic identity is preserved, including the significance of continued contact with others from the same ethnic group. As *Glazer and Moynihan* [1970] have so well shown, ethnicity continues as an important fact in contemporary social life across the adult years. The significance of aging in altering the meaning of ethnicity for personal and social adjustment requires additional study.

Contr. hum. Dev., vol. 14, pp. 80–85 (Karger, Basel 1985)

Families as Networks and Communities: A Developmental Psychology of Aging and Intergenerational Relations

Dean Rodeheaver

University of Wisconsin-Green Bay, Green Bay, Wisc., USA

Time plays a critical, though often understated, role in the functioning of families, social support networks, and communities. When we study intergenerational relations, we naturally consider changes in family function across time as individual family members face new developmental tasks. When we study social support networks, however, we do not consider as naturally the evolution of networks across the individual's life; rather, it often appears in our studies that networks emerge for the sole purpose of meeting specific life crises. I would like to illustrate the way the social networks of old people evolve over the course of their lives, just as family relationships evolve. In turn, I would like to suggest ways we might expand the study of intergenerational relations by addressing the impact of family functioning beyond the boundaries of the family – that is, its impact on social support networks and communities.

I will explore families as networks and communities using as my focus a question that fosters an evolutionary perspective: What are the consequences of living long, with the same people and often in the same place? This question arose from two investigations I conducted with rural elders in West Virginia. The first was a study of the social factors that influence the use of a public transportation program for the elderly. The second was an ethnography concerned with the maintenance of social status among elders in a rural church community. These studies suggest ways in which social aspects of aging as diverse as the use of social programs and the maintenance of community status are determined in part by intergenerational relations before the individual grows old.

Aging and Family History

West Virginia is a rural state in which transportation can be a major problem, particularly for the low-income elderly. In 1974 the state initiated a reduced-fare transportation stamp program (Transportation Remuneration Incentive Program – TRIP) for the low-income elderly and handicapped. Each month those eligible can purchase an $8.00 book of tickets for $3.00. These tickets can be used on any licensed and certified public vehicle – bus, taxi, train, or airplane.

An evaluation of the program conducted from 1975 to 1977 [Office of Research and Development, 1977] revealed that enrollment in the program had fallen far short of expectations: between 12 and 15% of those eligible for the program had actually enrolled. In addition to the usual problems associated with interventions of this kind, the evaluation revealed an excessive reliance on informal networks of transportation – transportation arrangements among friends, relatives, and neighbors.

In order to differentiate those who used the program from those who did not, I conducted in-depth exploratory interviews with 28 elderly individuals divided into three transportation style groups [Rodeheaver, 1981]. All the respondents used both informal networks and public transportation; they were grouped according to the degree to which they relied on each form of transportation. The first group included those who were enrolled in the program and used public transportation for most of their travel. The second group included individuals who were enrolled in the program but used public transportation less often than they rode with friends or relatives. The last group comprised individuals who were not enrolled in the program and used informal networks for most of their transportation.

The findings suggested that the groups did not differ with regard to availability of children, friends, or other people who could provide transportation. It was not uncommon, for example, to find a couple who relied on the bus, but whose children lived next door. Instead, the groups differed most in the length of time they had used informal transportation networks. The majority of those who relied primarily on informal networks had done so for more than 10 years. All of them had done so for at least 5 years. By contrast, the majority of those in the other groups had ridden with relatives and friends for only 1-5 years.

Within families, this difference reflects evolving intergenerational relations. One woman, for example, began to ride with her children as soon as they were old enough to drive, about 40 years ago. At the time of the interview, she was riding with her children and her grandchildren. Thus, for some of those who relied on informal networks, family transportation networks had not developed to meet the needs of an aging parent; they had developed to meet the needs of an entire family. Within these families, one could sense a continuity that was reflected in responses to questions about using public service programs in general. The individuals in these networks felt that such services may augment family care, but they certainly could not replace it. Many had not felt the need for service programs because 'The family has always been there'. Furthermore, those individuals would rather ask for help from other people than pay for it.

Within the other groups, however, family networks evolved differently. Individuals in these groups marked the beginning of their use of informal transportation networks with changes they associated with age: sudden illness, declining health, or the death of a spouse. They were no more likely to have experienced these changes, but the impact was different; they did not have the history of reliance on informal networks found in the group that used those networks most extensively. In addition, individuals in these two groups were more afraid of dependence, particularly on their children: As one man told me, 'We'd stay home all day rather than ask the kids for a ride.'

This difference in the evolution of family relations was further illustrated by the difference between those who relied on public transportation for most of their travel and those who used it to supplement their informal networks. The latter group had fewer children, relied on them less, and had larger potential networks – people with whom they did not ride, but could if they needed to. Thus, those who relied on public transportation were more likely to face the unwelcome prospect of dependence on their children, many of whom were no more financially secure than the elders were. Again, one can sense a continuity of life style and transportation style. Individuals who relied on public transportation had been using that form of transportation before the TRIP program began; the lower cost made the program very attractive. In addition, those individuals reported that public programs could replace family care and that they would rather pay for help than ask for it.

One of the consequences of living long with the same people, then, is that the practices, expectations, and attitudes one carries into old age have evolved over time. The evolution of these practices, expectations, and attitudes affects one's use of the resources available to meet the changes of aging.

Aging and Community History

The second study was an ethnographic exploration of the social status of elders in a rural church community, their psychological engagement in the community, and the resources they provided others. I conducted interviews with members of all but three of the elderly families in the church. In addition, I interviewed church members identified by the elderly as people who were important in their lives. Finally, I sent questionnaires to individuals who had joined the church within the past 5 years.

Responses indicated that the elders played significant roles in relationships with one another and maintained a relatively high social status ranking within the community. Four factors contributed to this status maintenance. First, there was a shared commitment by all church members to the future of the community. Second, the elders' continued attendance in church kept them visible to the congregation. Third, the elders had a recognized history of participation and leadership in the community. Fourth, the elders played a principle role in the history and traditions of the church. It is that historical role that I would like to develop further in this chapter.

The elders had strong family ties to the church. For example, some of the elders were descendants of the man who donated the land for the church. Many of the elders had attended the church all their lives and also represented the middle of five generations of church members – grandparents, parents, elders, children, and grandchildren. Consequently, their frequent reference to their 'family church' or their 'community church' was based on an association of as long as 140 years.

In addition, recent history has reinforced the status of the elders in the community. In 1974, the minister, with the support of the congregation, withdrew the church from the statewide Methodist church, leading to a legal battle over the church property. In the conflict that resulted, most of the congregation went elsewhere, leaving a core group of the elders and their families. Their commitment to their 'family church' was too strong for them to leave. After that, however, the church grew around the community of elders that remained, the elders remained active, and their children began to emerge as community leaders as well.

The status maintenance of the elders can be interpreted in part as an intergenerational flow of social credit – that is, a degree of social standing which permits a claim on community resources based on past rather than current activity [*Lozier and Althouse,* 1974, 1975]. The elders in this community had accumulated social credit during their own lives. Moreover, they were drawing on social credit that was established in previous generations, through the participation, leadership, and attendance of their parents and grandparents. Finally, to a smaller degree, they were drawing on the social credit that their children were beginning to accumulate as new leaders in the church. In addition to drawing on social credit, the elders had contributed to the social credit of their children, who anticipated growing old in the community in much the same way that their parents had.

Thus, one of the consequences of living long, with the same people, in the same place is that it permits the accumulation of social credit, not just over the course of the individual's life, but also across generations.

Conclusions

I have suggested that living long with the same people, and often in the same place, has important implications for intergenerational relations and for relations outside the family. The use of family networks early in life prepares one to meet the needs of aging with an established network. Family relations in communities contribute to the maintenance of social status through the accumulation of social credit across the life span and across generations.

Old people remain in close contact with their children throughout their lives and they also remain important to their children [*Troll* et al., 1979]. Furthermore, 44% of those over the age of 60 in 1970 had lived in the same house for at least 20 years; another 25% had lived in the same house for 10–20 years. Although mobility is increasing among the elderly, they are still not as mobile as other age groups, and when they do move, it is often within the same county [*Wiseman,* 1978]. Demographics suggest, then, that the consequences of a long life, with familiar people, in a familiar setting, are important for many old people.

An evolutionary perspective suggests important dimensions for social network analysis. Support networks do not arise spontaneously to meet crises. They accompany the individual across parts of the life course. How, then, do networks originate and why? Most important, how do they change as the developmental tasks, needs, and abilities of their members change? In addition, expanding the focus of intergenerational relations to include social networks and communities implies changes in social service programs. An evolutionary perspective, considering the flow of resources across the life span and across generations, assumes that unique histories create a variety of practices, expectations, and attitudes among elders. Consequently, the success of those programs is not guaranteed when they are directed at what is perceived as a homogeneous group of elders. Neither is the success of the new volunteerism. This perspective suggests that we not ask, 'Are there enough needy old people to support programs'; rather, we should ask, 'What do people need and when do they need it?'

Contr. hum. Dev., vol. 14, pp. 86–92 (Karger, Basel 1985)

Themes of Stability and Change in Grandparenting

Jeanne L. Thomas[a], *Nancy Datan*[b]

[a] University of Wisconsin-Parkside, Kenosha, and
[b] University of Wisconsin-Green Bay, Green Bay, Wisc., USA

In 1968, *Neugarten and Moore* noted that active parenting has become an experience primarily of early adulthood; a consequence is that grandparenting now potentially spans middle, as well as later, adulthood. Nonetheless, reviewers have noted that the nonspeculative literature on grandparenthood is scarce [e.g., *Troll,* 1980]. Developmental psychologists, furthermore, have repeatedly recognized the need to view grandparenting as an experience characterized by change [*Bengtson and Treas,* 1980; *Brody,* 1974; *Cohler and Grunebaum,* 1981; *Kivnick,* 1981, 1982a, b; *Troll and Bengtson,* 1979, 1982; *Wood and Robertson,* 1976]; however, empirical work in which change over time in grandparenting is examined has not followed these recommendations. In this study, we explored grandparents' perceptions of changes in relationships with grandchildren and their beliefs about the sources of these changes.

13 grandmothers and 6 grandfathers participated in the study. All had at least 2 grandchildren, and at least 1 grandchild living within 4 hours' travel; 15 grandparents had grandchildren living in their own community. Although they formed a small and nonrandom sample, the grandparents varied in demographic background (table I), as well as in length of grandparenting experience.

The senior author conducted a semistructured interview with each grandparent. Interview length ranged from 1½ to 3½ hours; interview topics included relationships with grandchildren, perceived changes in these

Table I. Demographic characteristics of the grandparents

	Grandmothers, n = 13	Grandfathers, n = 6
Mean age	58.9	69.7
Age range	52–70	63–78
Marital status		
Married	7	5
Widowed	4	1
Divorced	2	0
Education		
12 years or less	7	0
1–4 years college	5	3
Graduate degree	1	3
Annual family income		
Under $5,000	2	0
$6,000–10,000	3	0
$10,000–15,000	0	1
$16,000–20,000	1	3
$21,000–25,000	2	0
Over $26,000	5	2
Occupation		
Currently working	4	0
Retired	0	6
Full-time homemaker	9	0

relationships, and perceived sources of changes. Each tape-recorded interview was transcribed *verbatim,* and analyzed using thematic analysis. In the
thematic analysis, the senior author identified and described issues recurring within individual interviews and throughout the set of interviews. A
reliability judge reanalyzed a randomly selected sample of interview tran-
scripts; interjudge reliability was 0.93.

Two themes were identified. The first was a theme of stable aspects of
grandparenting; the second was a theme of discontinuity in this experience.
In describing both themes, we refer to grand*parents'* experiences, unless sex
differences in theme endorsement were identified.

Stability in Grandparenting

Respondents noted three types of stability in grandparenting. Grandparents' lack of parental responsibility for grandchildren, expectations about family assistance, and enjoyment of family companionship did not change over time.

Grandparents agreed that they did not have parental responsibility for grandchildren, and that this absence of responsibility was a basic part of being a grandparent. Grandmothers, but not grandfathers, explicitly distinguished parents' and grandparents' responsibilities. These women recognized that they had no need to make child-rearing decisions concerning appropriate behavior: grandmothers saw grandchildren during family visits, when their children handled misbehavior. Furthermore, grandmothers consciously and consistently distinguished between their own and their children's roles in grandchildren's care. One woman, for example, hesitated to feed her infant granddaughter for fear of detracting from the mother's time with the infant. A second woman refrained from advising adolescent grandchildren, since she believed that advising was a parental prerogative.

Grandfathers did not explicitly discuss boundaries of responsibility for grandchildren. However, men and women agreed that absence of responsibility was fundamental to their enjoyment of grandparenting. As Mr. Edwards (all names are pseudonyms) explained, 'when all of them are going hell-bent for election, I get sometimes upset, really ... that's one of the nice things about being a grandparent – you can ship them out, you know, when it gets too rough.'

A second source of continuity was the expectation of exchanging assistance within the family. Grandparents considered helping a familial obligation: they could depend upon relatives for help, and expected to aid children and grandchildren in any possible way. Mrs. Ferber explained that 'you feel like you're part of the family – being included' when grandchildren asked for help. Grandparents also believed that they had grown closer to children and grandchildren by helping. Mrs. Reed described her family with the statement that 'we're close now, we're all close – if one needs the other, we're here.' Similarly, Mr. Harding regretted his grandchildren's growing independence, which he viewed as a harbinger of distance in their relationship. Grandparents also enjoyed helping children and grandchildren. According to Mrs. Barry, 'all grandmothers would have to admit it – it's lovely to be needed!'

A third constant feature of grandparenting was enjoyment of family companionship. After grandchildren's birth, family gatherings were more frequent, and grandparents found their children's life-styles more compatible with their own. Mrs. Taylor, for example, reported more activities and vacations with her sons' families since grandchildren's birth: she explained that her sons' adoption of family-oriented habits made these occasions more frequent and more enjoyable. Grandparents also specifically valued grandchildren's companionship. Mr. Page, a retired widower, explained that 'I know people my age who don't have grandchildren, and they get along alright, but for me that's about all there is ...'

Grandparents emphasized the importance of family companionship in old age, as they expected familial bonds to be more enduring than ties outside the family. Grandparents of older children and adolescents most often voiced this expectation. However, grandparents of younger grandchildren uniformly hoped that they would remain close to their children and grandchildren.

Discontinuity in Grandparenting

The second theme comprised three areas of change in grandparenting. Grandparents viewed relationships with grandchildren as undergoing continual transformation through grandchildren's maturation. Grandparents also noted changes in patterns of intergenerational assistance; these changes were related to grandchildren's growth and to the maturation of children's families. Finally, grandparents contrasted their absence of parental responsibility for grandchildren with the greater responsibility that they had felt as parents.

Grandparents agreed that relationships with grandchildren had changed over time, and that these changes stemmed primarily from grandchildren's development. As grandchildren acquired new interests and abilities, activities during family visits changed. One man explained that 'they're pretty much the ones who gauge what is done, because you'd have a heck of a time getting them to do things that they don't want to do. So they pretty much dictate.'

Changes over time in sources of satisfaction in grandparenting also reflected grandchildren's development. Grandparents enjoyed observing the expansion of grandchildren's capabilities and personalities; they also noted that activities with grandchildren that they especially liked were only possible, practical, or enjoyable when the children had attained a particular maturational level. Mrs. Lane, for example, most enjoyed cuddling, which the children resisted after infancy, and adult conversation and companionship, which had not been possible until her older grandchildren reached adolescence. Similarly, grandparents explained changes in stresses of grandparenting as consequences of grandchildren's development. As grandchildren grew from dependent infants to more autonomous preschoolers, they also became more disobedient; many grandparents were annoyed at grandchildren's disobedience. The elementary school years brought greater compliance; however, compliance was followed by renewed defiance, and renewed stress for grandparents, during adolescence.

A few grandparents also noted or anticipated the impact of their own development. Mr. Gage increasingly relied upon his young adult grandchildren for assistance, as his own physical strength declined; Mrs. Barry anticipated a similar change, remarking that she might someday find that decreased agility constrained activities with grandchildren. Mrs. Caine was unable to continue the outings with grandchildren that she had enjoyed prior to her husband's death, since her finances were now limited and since she did not drive.

A second type of change in grandparenting was in the pattern of intergenerational assistance. During the formative years of children's families, grandparents provided assistance. Young grandchildren 'helped' with tasks and errands, but grandparents delegated these duties more to occupy the grandchild than to establish reciprocity; grandparents did not report receiving help from their own children at this time. However, grandparents of older children, adolescents, and young adults described a mutual flow of assistance: grandchildren were cooperative and capable helpers, and grandparents said that they received help from their own children. At the same time, these grandparents assisted their children and grandchildren.

The final aspect of discontinuity was a perceived contrast between parents' and grandparents' responsibilities. Earlier, we discussed grandparents' absence of responsibility for grandchildren's upbringing as a type of stability. However, most grandparents, in describing this lack of responsibility, contrasted their current situation with their earlier parental experience. Mrs. Barry explained that 'it is totally different ... you know that whatever you do with the child, you first have to ask the parent. The decision-making power that you had with your own children ... it isn't there, because you're not the parent.' When considered in the context of respondents' family-life cycle experience, grandparents' absence of parental responsibility reflected discontinuity.

To review, we have described two themes of grandparenting. The first was a theme of stability, comprising descriptions of absence of parental responsibility for grandchildren, feelings about family assistance, and enjoyment of family companionship. The second theme concerned discontinuity in grandparenting, and included descriptions of changes in relationships with grandchildren, differences in intergenerational assistance patterns, and a perceived contrast between parents' and grandparents' responsibilities.

Discussion and Conclusion

In considering the study findings, we offer two conclusions. First, we agree that a developmental perspective of intergenerational relations and of grandparenting is needed; such an approach calls for complex empirical approaches to intergenerational relations. Our findings suggest that investigators must consider multiple dimensions of change (e.g., in shared activities, in satisfactions, in assistance patterns, in sources of stress) and examine multiple determinants of each change dimension (e.g., development of each relationship partner, the family life cycle). In addition, the researcher must decide upon a context or contexts (e.g., experience in a particular relationship, family experiences throughout the life span, ethnic traditions) within which to examine change dimensions and their determinants.

Our second conclusion is that, even as researchers attempt to achieve a developmental perspective of intergenerational relations, the stable characteristics of these relationships must not be overlooked. In this study, grandparents described aspects of relationships with grandchildren which did not change over time, as well as areas in which changes were apparent. One might consider these stable facets to be subjective defining characteristics of grandparenting, or fundamental parts of grandparent identity; additional study of these features would enhance our understanding of grandparenting and of intergenerational relations in general. For example, researchers might consider whether similar constant features are apparent in other family relationships and/or friendships of later life; individual and ethnic group differences in stable characteristics of intergenerational relations should also be considered.

This study had as a focus the issue of temporal change and stability in grandparenting; however, the study addressed only a few of many important questions in this area. Consequences of historical change for grandparenting and for other intergenerational experiences require additional study; furthermore, the impact of intergenerational experiences on individual development, particularly in adulthood, should be clarified. As scholars explore these areas, a life-span developmental model of intergenerational relations will become a more realizable goal.

Contr. hum. Dev., vol. 14, pp. 93–109 (Karger, Basel 1985)

Intergenerational Relations:
Personal Meaning in the Life Cycle

Helen Q. Kivnick

University of California, Berkeley, Calif., and
University of Pennsylvania, Philadelphia, Pa., USA

The nature and importance of intergenerational relations in our society are influenced by such sociodemographic shifts as increased life expectancy, changes in the timing and patterning of the family cycle, changes in the rates of divorce and remarriage, changes in sex roles, and changes in work life [*Hagestad,* 1983; *Hareven,* 1977; *Treas and Bengtson,* 1982]. In particular, the shift toward a decreasing proportion of adult life being spent in active parenting, in the context of a life expectancy which now approaches 80 years, is recognized as exerting a profound effect on relations across the generations. When women bore children throughout their years of fertility, it was not at all unusual for parents to become grandparents while they were still actively involved in raising young children and, not infrequently, in bearing infants. The behavior and meaning of grandparenthood under such family circumstances may be expected to have differed markedly from those of today's grandparents for whom, by and large, grandparenthood succeeds active parenting rather than accompanying it.

Alongside these shifts in family timing and patterning, the expectability of long life carries with it the expectation that intergenerational relationships will endure for decades [*Hagestad,* 1981]. In an era in which the life expectancy approaches 80 years, parents in their 40s and their adult children over 20 may reasonably expect to relate to one another as adults for another 30 to 40 years, or longer. The rewards and burdens of these long-term bonds, the shared experiences accumulated, the patterns of reciprocal influence, caring, and assistance developed, and the larger generational context in which these bonds develop – all of these factors determine the meaning this kind of intergenerational relationship will hold for its participants. A couple whose first grandchild is born when they are 45 can reasonably expect to be the grandparents of that child for 30–35 years or longer, through his or her early and middle adulthood. Thus grandparenthood, too, becomes a relationship which a given dyad of grandparent and grandchild may expect to share for nearly half a lifetime. This relationship will hold individual, personal meaning for grandparent and for grandchild. This meaning will influence and be influenced by a multiplicity of factors having to do with the developmental stage, cohort, personality, health, work status, family constellation, socioeconomic status, etc. of grandparent and grand-child – and with changes in all of these factors over the years.

Clearly the phenomenon of intergenerational relations is complex, intertwined as it is with historical developments in society and demography, on one hand, and with intricacies of individual personality and development, on the other. Indeed, even the term 'intergenerational relations' is less than straightforward, referring to a wide variety of relationships among individuals at all stages of the life cycle. Within the family, intergenerational relations include all relationships between persons who are not of the same lineage 'tier' [*Hagestad,* 1983]. These relationships may exist between contiguous generations, e.g., parent and child, and also across generations which are differentially noncontiguous, e.g., grandparent and grandchild, great grandparent and great grandchild, etc.

People participate, filially, in the contiguous intergenerational relationship of parenthood from the moment that they are born, until the moment that their parents have died. (Indeed, it may be argued that we remain psychodynamically involved with our parents until we, ourselves, have died.) People participate in this relationship, parentally, from the first moment that they become parents. We are grandchildren at least as long as our grandparents remain alive; we are grandparents from the birth of our first grandchild. We may participate in many intergenerational relationships at the same time. For example, as a function of current patterns of family timing and life expectancy, a woman in her 40s may realistically expect, simultaneously, to be the daughter to living parents, the grand-daughter to one or more aged grandparents, the mother to children, and the grandmother to young grandchildren. Though any one individual's relationship partners (specific persons) and relationship roles (e.g., grandchild and grandparent) change over the course of the life cycle, participation in these intergenerational relations, themselves, is likely to persist, in some form, from birth until death. If for no reason other than their normative duration throughout vast segments of the life cycle, these intergenerational relationships must be regarded as relevant to development throughout life.

Understanding them and their meaning to members of all generations can contribute immeasurably to our understanding of development at every phase of the life cycle.

To my knowledge we do not yet have a succinct, standardized terminology for differentiating readily among various kinds of intergenerational relations. At least for purposes of this chapter, I shall use the descriptor 'cross-generational' to refer to relationships such as grandparenthood, between individuals of noncontiguous generations.

Psychosocial Development in the Life Cycle

The body of this chapter will discuss the meaning of intergenerational relations in terms of psychosocial development in the life cycle. In particular, I shall focus on the role of grandparenthood, one cross-generational relationship, in the psychosocial development of older adults. This discussion is based on the Erikson eight-stage model of the life cycle [*Erikson,* 1950; 1982], and draws heavily on research currently being conducted by *E. Erikson, J. Erikson,* and myself to elaborate and clarify this model. The Eriksons' model suggests that in the course of living a life, the individual grows through a sequence of eight stages. It is my understanding that these stages are not proposed as conforming to the strict requirements of developmental stage theory. Rather, I view them as constructs which enable us to understand shifts in psychosocial focus and continuities in psychosocial dynamics over the life cycle of any given individual. Perhaps the word 'phase' is more appropriate to such a construct. Each of these eight phases is characterized by a focal psychosocial tension between two opposites; dynamically balancing these two opposites is regarded as the focal psychosocial challenge of the phase. For example, the phase of middle adulthood is said to be characterized by a tension between the sense of Generativity and the sense of Stagnation. Each individual's middle adulthood is viewed, in these terms, as focusing on a struggle to balance Generative expressions (e.g., creativity, procreativity, productivity [*Erikson,* 1980]) with expressions of Stagnation (e.g., relaxing, focusing on oneself, taking time out, or, in California, laying back and mellowing out). The actual process of balancing a psychosocial tension is largely unconscious. However, this unconscious, internal process is made possible by the behavioral, cognitive, and affective expressions we regard as comprising a life. That is, internal, psychodynamic work takes place in a meaningful fashion only in the context of the individual's vital involvement with the people, materials, institutions, and experiences that make up the society in which he or she lives.

With unfortunate regularity, the Erikson formulation is misunderstood as saying that at any phase the individual is entirely absorbed by the psychosocial challenge which is currently focal. This misunderstanding implies that by the end of each phase, the individual must have resolved the focal challenge in order to have the wherewithal to meet the challenge of the next phase. The next mistaken implication is that in any phase the individual's ability to achieve a successful resolution of the focal challenge is predetermined and foreclosed by the cumulative success of earlier resolutions. Central to correcting this series of misunderstandings is what we are currently calling the principle of renewing and previewing (or, perhaps, reworking and preworking). According to this principle, the individual is involved in renewing earlier psychosocial balances, and in previewing, as it were, those psychosocial tensions which have yet to become focal. (And remember that the processes of renewing and previewing, like that of struggling to balance a tension between two opposites, are internal, largely unconscious concomitants of more visible behavioral expressions.) These processes of renewing and previewing take place regardless of whether or not a given age-appropriate resolution was adequate. They take place alongside the struggle to balance whatever psychosocial tension is currently focal, and are, in a very real way, part and parcel of balancing the focal tension. (The complexity of these concepts makes them difficult to summarize. They have been discussed at somewhat greater length by this author [*Kivnick, 1983b*], and they will be discussed fully in a manuscript by *E. Erikson, J. Erikson,* and myself that is currently in preparation. I have provided this summary at the present time, because these concepts comprise an essential foundation for my discussion of the function of cross-generational relations for people in later life.)

I do not mean to suggest that the psychosocial phases and their focal tensions represent rigid cells into which we must classify behaviors and feelings in order to account completely for a life. I see no inherent value in such accounting. We are using terms such as 'psychosocial tension' and 'Integrity versus Despair' as keywords for or condensations of complex concepts which we have found to be useful in organizing an integrated understanding of the life cycle. We are perpetually revising these concepts to conform to our data. (I trust that we are also prepared to abandon these concepts, should others emerge as more useful.)

In terms of this life cycle formulation, the individual whose focal challenge is to balance a sense of Integrity with that of Despair is *also,* simultaneously, involved in renewing balances for earlier tensions. As a relationship that is available to most older adults, grandparenthood provides a context within which much essential renewing, reviewing, and reworking can take place. In these terms, the ambiguity surrounding the behaviors, rights, and responsibilities of grandparenthood [*Hagestad,* 1983; *Troll,* 1983; *Hess and Waring,* 1978; *Kivnick,* 1982c; *Wood,* 1982] does not diminish the developmental value of this relationship. However, this ambiguity does render such value highly individualized, rather than uniform or institutionalized.

As a point of reference, let us consider parenthood and middle adulthood. For all of its contemporary variability, parenthood is generally recognized as involving a parent's responsibility for certain amounts of protection, nurturance, and socialization of the child. Fulfilling these responsibilities is readily understandable as valuable to the parent's internal struggle to balance Generativity and Stagnation. Thus, whether we regard parenthood as the key to the life cycle [*Gutmann,* 1975] or simply as a normative role in adulthood, we can easily recognize it as closely related, behaviorally, to essential psychosocial development in adulthood.

Considerations of later adulthood and old age become far more complex. The tremendous interindividual variability that characterizes all aspects of this period makes it difficult to identify meaningful, unifying psychosocial themes, or the normative roles and behaviors we may expect to be associated with such themes. It has been suggested that an accurate formulation of the entire life cycle must incorporate at least one additional phase – perhaps focusing on development among the young old, or perhaps focusing on the deterioration which frequently succeeds mature wisdom. Our data do not seem to suggest the existence of two or three identifiable, universal phases after middle adulthood. However, they *do* indicate that psychosocial development after the period of direct responsibility for 'the maintenance of the world' [*Erikson,* 1980] must focus on a challenge more substantial than coming to terms with the life that has already been lived. We suggest that, at least for the moment, a broad conceptualization of the struggle to balance Integrity and Despair is, in fact, a useful way to think about the psychodynamic underpinnings of that part of the life cycle which succeeds the period of direct maintenance responsibility in multifarious spheres. We also suggest that participation in cross-generational relationships is a form of involvement which can be invaluable in developing a healthy balance in the process of this struggle.

Grandparenthood Meaning

Each individual life is part of various, interlocking networks of lives, included among which is the family generational cycle. In living through later adulthood, the grandparent is inextricably involved in the middle adulthood of the parent generation, in the adolescence or childhood of grandchildren, and perhaps in the childhood of great-grandchildren and the very old age of his or her parents, as well. These cross-generational involvements affect the quality of psychosocial development of all participants. For grandchildren, for example, relationships with grandparents exert an influence on the particular kind of balance the child will be able to manage, for each age-appropriate psychosocial tension. Let us consider the following preschool-aged girl. Her father's work requires him to travel a good deal, and her mother goes with him whenever possible. This girl spends at least 2 weeks of every month living with her grandparents. Her current relationship with her parents is experienced as a succession of tearful partings and joyful reunions. When her parents are home they are so glad to be with her that they seem to delight in everything she does. They make few attempts at discipline, allowing her to behave largely according to impulse and to play with any object which catches her fancy. They do not restrict her behavior according to potential danger to child or property. Instead they most often swoop in at the last moment, either rescuing their daughter from imminent harm, or comforting her after the damage has been done.

For this child it is the grandparents with whom she learns to balance Initiative and Guilt. It is they who show consistent pleasure at certain kinds of behaviors and consistent displeasure at others. It is they who follow through on her curiosity, attempting to help her answer questions. It is they who delight in her enthusiasm while teaching her to curb her exuberance. This girl's early senses of Initiative and Guilt are forever linked to the Irish couple in their 50s who are her grandparents. Her early sense of Purpose is built around her grandfather's love of singing and her grandmother's love of the Church. These early factors will undoubtedly undergo many transformations as this child grows up, but their initial form and the role they play in her age-appropriate sense of Purpose are undeniable effects of her relationship with her grandparents.

In a reciprocal fashion, relationships with grandchildren facilitate the grandparent's essential psychodynamic work on the psychosocial tasks that are central to what I shall call 'postmaintenance adulthood'. Let us consider the grandparents mentioned above. These people have launched all of their children, and they are proud and satisfied with 'the job we did as parents. They're all on their own now and they don't look to us for every little thing. Of course we're still involved, but we're not responsible in the same way.' This notion of being 'not responsible in the same way' is central to what I have been referring to as renewing the balance between Generativity and Stagnation in the postmaintenance phase. As the grandmother says, 'My family has always been my life. My family and the Church. It's always been my job to take care of them, all their little wants and wishes, and teach them to love the Lord. In a way I'm out of a job now, which is why I'm so glad to have each little grandchild whenever they want to come. In another way, my job now is different. I can wait on my husband like a king, and I haven't done that since before my first one was born. I can think, maybe a little bit, about whether I might like to have a new couch or a new dress, or stop in the middle of the day to have coffee with a friend. I can watch my own children being parents. See what they learned from all my teaching. See what I'd do different if I had to raise 'em today. With the grandchildren I just fill in the gaps. Sometimes I think all I have to do with them is enjoy them. But my husband says I couldn't stop teaching things to children if my life depended on it. In a way, now, I have to be more careful – not to get in the way of how the parents raise their children, but still making sure that these little grandchildren pick up what I know is important. In another way I don't have to worry at all. It's not my responsibility any more. I can do whatever feels right with the grandchildren, help out the parents where I can, and mostly sit back and feel proud of this family my husband and I have raised. I can hardly believe they're all grown up!'

This woman is describing various aspects of postmaintenance Generativity. Her main life task is no longer to nurture her children and to teach them essential values. In grandparenthood, she finds herself experimenting with many of the components of her mothering role. To some extent, she feels displaced, with no object for her caretaking skills. In these terms, she uses time with her grandchildren as an opportunity to continue to exercise these skills. She finds herself caring for her husband in new ways, and she is beginning to pay new attention to her own pleasures, i.e., to care for herself in new ways. She recognizes that postmaintenance parenthood is different from maintenance-phase parenthood. Rather than actively shaping and molding her children, she can watch them with their own children, regarding their adulthood behaviors as a kind of evaluation of her success in raising them, 20 to 30 years ago. She is eager to see her children do well, both because she wants them to be happy and also because their success reflects well on her. She enjoys assisting them in whatever ways seem appropriate. She struggles not to interfere with their parenting, but she also feels obliged to make sure there are no crucial gaps in her grandchildren's upbringing. She is relieved not to be burdened with the responsibilities of parenthood, but her level of ongoing involvement with her children and their families means that she is not free of concern. She is not responsible for active parenting, either for her children or for her grandchildren; neither is she free from responsibility to them. Clarifying the nature of this postmaintenance responsibility and expressing it with Integrity is an essential component of renewing Generativity versus Stagnation in postmaintenance adulthood. Of course this process is broader and more inclusive than discussed thus far. I have used the preceding example simply as an illustration of the way grandparenthood and its role behaviors and meanings can facilitate various dimensions of this age-appropriate, psychodynamic process.

The plethora of meanings and behaviors that researchers have identified as inherent in grandparenthood may be understood as facilitating the grandparent's renewing age-appropriate balances for many earlier psychosocial tensions, not simply that between Generativity and Stagnation. For example, grandparenthood in terms of mutual love and security, as discussed by *Benedek* [1970], *Blau* [1973], and *Boyd* [1969], may be understood as part of the grandparent's renewing an age-appropriate sense of Intimacy. To the extent that mutual love and security are part of the meaning of grandparenthood for a given grandparent, interactions with grandchildren provide occasions for experiencing these essential feelings. Every relationship in which these feelings play a part provides an opportunity for this grandparent to renew an age-appropriate balance around the earlier tension between Intimacy and Isolation. This tension has to do with feelings of love and mutuality, with relationship partners in all generations. For some postmaintenance adults, freedom from maintenance responsibilities may provide a new opportunity for mutuality in relationships. Mutuality across generations is different from mutuality within the same generation, but both are part of balancing Intimacy with Isolation in postmaintenance adulthood. This period is likely to involve many adults in caretaking responsibilities for their elderly parents. For these individuals, love and mutuality in grandparenthood must exist alongside caring for the middle-generation parents with whom love and mutuality must now take new forms. Regardless of the relationship context, however, the mutual love and security described as inherent in grandparenthood provide many grandparents an array of experiences and feelings which contribute to these individuals' later-life struggle to renew an age-appropriate balance between Intimacy and Isolation.

Other identified meanings of grandparenthood may be discussed in a similar fashion. Grandparenthood in terms of authority and responsibility [*Kahana and Kahana,* 1971] or freedom therefrom [*Albrecht,* 1954; *Apple,* 1956] may be understood in terms of renewing age-appropriate Generativity versus Stagnation. The dimension of grandparenthood meaning I identified as *Immortality through Clan* [*Kivnick,* 1982a, b; 1983a] may be understood as renewing the essential senses of Hope and Faith. The dimension I have referred to as *Indulgence* would seem to be closely related to themes of competence and care. The very poignance of grandparenthood ambiguity may be understood as part of the postmaintenance adult's age-appropriate reinvolvement with struggles between Identity and Identity Confusion and with Industry and Inferiority. To the extent that the grandparent is good for grandchildren and middle-generation parents, i.e., to the extent that the grandparent facilitates psychosocial well-being in members of younger generations – to that extent the grandparent has been effective in a dimension of renewing his or her own sense of Generativity. This list of examples is far from exhaustive. Rather, it is intended to illustrate some of the ways that grandparenthood, as discussed by social scientists, may be seen as an integral part of the psychosocial processes of postmaintenance adulthood.

Grandparenthood Behaviors

There are tremendous individual differences in the meaning of particular behaviors. That is, the same behavior is likely to represent a variety of different meanings to different individuals [*Kivnick,* 1983c, 1984]. Therefore a discussion of grandparenthood behaviors, per se, would be likely to tell us little about the diversity of meanings this role holds, both across and within individuals. A similar diversity exists in the kinds of internal dynamics associated, across individuals, with a particular issue. Let us consider the effort to balance Generativity and Stagnation, during the phase of active maintenance. Some people express nurturant parenting with little conflict, finding easy satisfaction in meeting the needs of growing children. Other people are frightened by the realistic helplessness and dependence of children. While they meet their children's essential physical needs, they may be unable to provide consistent nurturance and dependability. Some parents must struggle to find time and energy for their own sustenance, in the face of the perceived demands of small children. Others must struggle to subordinate their own wishes, if they are to provide more than superficial care for their growing children. Although we can meaningfully discuss psychosocial tensions across subjects, the specific dynamics of any one tension are unique to each individual. In a similar fashion, the dynamics of renewing psychosocial balances, of reworking earlier psychosocial tensions, may be expected to be unique to each individual. A behavior which has to do primarily with age-appropriate issues of Intimacy for one grandparent might be more closely linked with issues of Competence or Generativity for another. Thus, we cannot identify particular behaviors as universally linked to the renewing of specific psychosocial tensions. Society could impose universal, behavioral rights and responsibilities on the grandparent role. Even then, however, the psychosocial meanings of any specific behavior would vary across grandparents.

In the social pluralism of contemporary America, belaboring the grandparenthood relationship in terms of role requirements or the lack thereof does not seem likely to enhance our understanding of the meaning of grandparenthood, either to grandparents or to members of other generations. However, considering this cross-generational relationship in terms of its psychosocial role in the concluding phase of the life cycle does promise to contribute both to our understanding of grandparenthood, and also to our understanding of postmaintenance life as a whole. To this end I reiterate that grandparenthood seems to facilitate the grandparent's involvement in various of the psychosocial tasks of postmaintenance adulthood. If we can begin to consider large-scale, survey-research findings in these individual, qualitative, psychodynamic terms, perhaps we can begin to make meaningful progress toward understanding the process of living an integrated, postmaintenance life as an individual, in a family, in a society, and in history.

Contr. hum. Dev., vol. 14, pp. 103–110 (Karger, Basel 1985)

References Symposium Articles

Abramson, H.: Ethnic diversity in Catholic America (Wiley Interscience, New York 1973).

Alba, R.: Social assimilation among American Catholic national origin groups. Am. sociol. Rev. *41:* 1030–1046 (1976).

Alba, R.: The twilight of ethnicity among American Catholics of European ancestry. Ann. Am. Ass. polit. soc. Sci. *454:* 86–97 (1981).

Albrecht, R.: The parental responsibilities of grandparents. Marr. Fam. Living *16:* 201–204 (1954).

Apple, D.: The social structure of grandparenthood. Am. Anthrop. *58:* 656–663 (1956).

Arensberg, C.; Kimball, S.: Family and community in Ireland (Harvard University Press, Cambridge 1968).

Baltes, P.; Cornelius, S.; Nesselroade, J.: Cohort effects in developmental psychology; in Nesselroade, Baltes, Longitudinal research in the study of behavior and development (Academic Press, New York 1979).

Banfield, E.: The moral basis of a backward society (Macmillan/Free Press, New York 1958).

Baron, M.: People who intermarry: intermarriage in a New England industrial community (Syracuse University Press, Syracuse 1946).

Barth, J.: Introduction; in Barth, Ethnic groups and boundaries: the social organization of culture differences (Little, Brown, Boston 1969).

Benedek, T.: Parenthood during the life cycle; in Anthony, Benedek, Parenthood during the life cycle (Little, Brown, Boston 1970).

Benedict, R.: Chrysanthemum and the sword: patterns of Japanese culture (Houghton Mifflin, Boston 1946).

Bengtson, V.L.; Cutler, N.E.: Generations and intergenerational relations: perspectives on age groups and social change; in Binstock, Shanas, Handbook of aging and the social sciences (Van Nostrand Reinhold, New York 1976).

Bengtson, V.L.; Dowd, J.; Smith, D.; Inkeles, A.: Modernization, modernity, and perceptions of aging: a cross-cultural study. J. Geront. *30:* 688–695 (1975).

Bengtson, V.L.; Treas, J.: The changing family context of mental health and aging; in Birren, Sloan, Handbook of mental health and aging (Prentice Hall, Englewood Cliffs 1980).

Bianco, C.: The two rosetos (Indiana University Press, Bloomington, 1974).

Biddle, E.: The American Catholic Irish family; in Mindel, Habenstein, Ethnic families in America (Elsevier, New York 1976).

Blalock, H.: Toward a theory of minority group relations (Wiley, New York 1967).

Blau, Z.S.: Old age in a changing society (Franklin Watts, New York 1973).

Boissevain, J.: Poverty and politics in a Sicilian agro-town. Int. J. Ethnogr. *1:* 198–236 (1966).

Botwinick, J.: Intellectual abilities; in Birren, Schaie, Handbook of the psychology of aging (Van Nostrand Reinhold, New York 1977).

Boyd, R.R.: The valued grandparent: a changing social role; in Donahue, Kornbluh, Power, Living in the multigenerational family (Institute of Gerontology, University of Michigan, Ann Arbor 1969).

Brody, E.M.: Aging and family personality: a developmental view. Fam. Process *13:* (1974).

Brubaker, T.H.: Family relationships in later life (Sage Publications, Beverly Hills 1983).

Chance, N.: Acculturation, self-identification, and personality adjustment. Am. Anthrop. *67:* 372–393 (1965).

Chown, S.: Age and the rigidities. J. Geront. *16:* 353–362 (1961).

Chown, S.: Personality and aging. Unpublished manuscript (West Virginia University, Morgantown 1968).

Clark, M.: Cultural values and dependency in later life; in Cowgill, Holmes, Aging and modernization (Appleton-Century-Crofts, New York 1972).

Cohen, C.: The lesson of ethnicity; in Cohen, Urban ethnicity (Tavistock Publications, London 1974).

Cohler, B.: Autonomy and interdependence in the family of adulthood: a psychological perspective. Gerontologist *23:* 33–39 (1983).

Cohler, B.; Grunebaum, H.: Mothers, grandmothers, and daughters (Wiley, New York 1981).

Cohler, B.; Lieberman, M.: Ethnicity and personal adaptation. Int. J. Group Tensions *7:* 20–41 (1977/1978).

Devereux, G.: Ethnic identity: its logical functions and its dysfunctions; in De Vos, Romanucci-Ross, Ethnic identity: cultural continuities and change (Mayfield Publishing, Palo Alto 1975).

Dobrowski, L.: Poland; in Palmore, International handbook on aging (Greenwood Press, Westport 1980).

Easterlin, R.: Immigration: economic and social characteristics; in Threnstrom, Harvard encyclopedia of American ethnic groups (Harvard University Press, Cambridge 1980).

Erikson, E.H.: On the generational cycle: an address. Int. J. Psycho-Analysis *61:* 213–233 (1980).

Erikson, E.H.: The life cycle completed (Norton, New York 1982).

Erikson, E.H.; Erikson, J.M.: Growth and crises of the 'health personality'; in Milton, Symposium on the health personality (Josiah Macy Jr. Found., New York 1950).

Etzioni, A.: The ghetto: a re-evaluation. Social Forces *37:* 255–262 (1959).

Fandetti, D.; Gelfand, D.: Care of the aged: attitudes of white ethnic families. Gerontologist *16:* 544–549 (1976).

Femminella, F.; Quadagno, J.: The Italian-American family; in Mindel, Habenstein, Ethnic families in America: patterns and variations (Elsevier, New York 1976).

Fleetwood, J.: Ireland; in Palmore, International handbook on aging: contemporary developments and research (Greenwood Press, Westport 1980).

Florea, A.: Italy; in Palmore, International handbook on aging: contemporary developments and research (Greenwood Press, Westport 1980).

Fogel, R.W.; Hatfield, E.; Kiesler, S.B.; Shanas, E.: Aging: stability and change in the family (Academic Press, New York 1981).

Fried, M.: The world of the urban working class (Harvard University Press, Cambridge 1973).

Galtung, J.: Members of two worlds (Columbia University Press, New York 1971).

Gans, H.: The urban villagers (Free Press, New York 1962).

Gelfand, D.: Aging: the ethnic factor (Little, Brown, Boston 1982).

Gelfand, D.; Fandetti, D.: Suburban and urban white ethnics: attitudes towards care of the aged. Gerontologist 20: 588–594 (1980).

Glazer, N.; Moynihan, D.: Beyond the melting pot (MIT Press, Cambridge 1970).

Gleason, P.: American identity and Americanization; in Thernstrom, Harvard encyclopedia of American ethnic groups (Harvard University Press, Cambridge 1980).

Golab, C.: The immigrant and the city: Poles, Italians and Jews in Philadelphia; in Davis, Haller, The peoples of Philadelphia (Temple University Press, Philadelphia 1973).

Gordon, M.: Assimilation in American life: the role of race, religion, and ethnic origins (Oxford University Press, New York 1964).

Gordon, M.: Human nature, class and ethnicity (Oxford University Press, New York 1978).

Gorer, G.; Rickman, J.: The people of Great Russia (Cressat Press, London 1950).

Greeley, A.: Ethnicity as an influence on behavior; in Feinstein, Ethnic groups in the city (Heath, Lexington 1971).

Greeley, A.: The most distressful nation: the taming of the Irish (Quadrangle Books, Chicago 1972).

Greeley, A.: Ethnicity in the United States: a preliminary reconnaissance (Wiley Interscience, New York 1974).

Greeley, A.; McCready, W.: The transmission of cultural heritages: the case of the Irish and the Italians; in Glazer, Moynihan, Ethnicity: theory and experience (Harvard University Press, Cambridge 1975).

Gutmann, D.: Parenthood: key to the comparative study of the life-cycle; in Datan, Ginsburg, Life-span developmental psychology: normative life crises (Academic Press, New York 1975).

Gutmann, D.: The cross-cultural perspective: notes toward a comparative psychology of aging; in Birren, Schaie, Handbook of the psychology of aging (Van Nostrand Reinhold, New York 1977).

Hagestad, G.O.: Problems and promises in the social psychology of intergenerational relations; in Fogel, Hatfield, Kilser, Marck, Aging: stability and change in the family (Academic Press, New York 1981).

Hagestad, G.O.: Grandparenthood and intergenerational processes: continuity and connectedness. National Conference on Grandparenthood, Wingspread, Wisc. 1983.

Handlin, O.: The uprooted (Atlantic Monthly Press/Little, Brown, Boston 1951).

Handlin, O.: Race and nationality in American life (Little Brown, Boston 1957).

Hansen, M.: The problem of the third-generation immigrant. Presented to the Augustana, Illinois Historical Society, 1938.

Hansen, M.: The Atlantic migration, 1607–1860 (Havard University Press, Cambridge 1940).

Hansen, M.: The third generation in America. Commentary *14:* 492–500 (1952).

Hareven, T.K.: Family time and historical time. Daedalus *106:* 57–70 (1977).

Hareven, T.; Modell, J.: Family patterns; in Thernstrom, Harvard encyclopedia of American ethnic groups (Havard University, Press, Cambridge 1980).

Hess, B.B.; Waring, J.M.: Parent and child in later life: rethinking the relationship; in Lerner, Spanier, Child influences on marital and family interaction (Academic Press, New York 1978).

Heiss, J.: Residential segregation and the assimilation of Italians in an Australian city. Int. Migrat. Rev. *4:* 165–171 (1966).

Inkeles, A.: Personality and social structure; in Merton, Broom, Cottrell, Sociology today: problems and prospects (Basic Books, New York 1961).

Inkeles, A.; Levinson, D.: National character: the study of modal personality and sociocultural systems; in Lindzey, Handbook of social psychology, vol. II (Addison-Wesley, Reading 1954).

Kahana, E.; Kahana, B.: Theoretical and research perspectives on grandparenthood. Aging hum. Dev. *2:* 261–268 (1971).

Kantowicz, E.: Polish-American politics in Chicago (University of Chicago Press, Chicago 1975).

Kardiner, A.: The psychological frontiers of society (Columbia University Press, New York 1945).

Kemper, R.: Migration and adaptation: Tzintzuntzan peasants in Mexico City (Sage Publications, Beverly Hills 1977).

Kennedy, R.: Single or triple melting pot? Intermarriage trends in New Haven. Am. J. Sociol. *49:* 331–339 (1944) or *58:* 56–59 (1952).

Kivnick, H.Q.: Grandparenthood and the mental health of grandparents. Ageing Soc. *1:* 365–391 (1981).

Kivnick, H.Q.: Grandparenthood: an overview of meaning and mental health. Gerontologist *22:* 59–66 (1982a).

Kivnick, H.Q.: The meaning of grandparenthood (UMI Research Press, Ann Arbor 1982b).

Kivnick, H.Q.: Dimensions of grandparenthood meaning: deductive conceptualization and empirical derivation. J. Pers. soc. Psychol. *44:* 1056–1068 (1983a).

Kivnick, H.Q.: Integrity vs. despair: the final stage reconsidered. Presented at Symposium conducted in collaboration with Erik H. Erikson and Joan M. Erikson: The life cycle revisited (University of Pennsylvania, Department of Psychiatry, Philadelphia, Pa. 1983b).

Kivnick, H.Q.: Grandparenthood and other life processes: discussion of a paper by Lillian Troll. Presented at National Conference on Grandparenthood, Wingspread, Wisc. 1983c).

Kivnick, H.Q.: Grandparents and family relations; in Quinn, Hughston, Independent aging: perspectives in social gerontology (Aspen Systems Corp., Rockville 1984).

Kluckhohn, C.: Values and value orientation; in Parsons, Toward a general theory of action (Harvard University Press, Cambridge 1951).

Kluckhohn, C.: Mirror for man: a survey of human behavior and social attitudes (Fawcett Publications, Greenwich 1959).

Kluckhohn, C.; Strodtbeck, F.: Variations in value orientation (Harper & Row, New York 1961).

Kolm, R.: Ethnicity in society and community; in Feinstein, Ethnic groups in the city: culture, institutions, and power (Heath, Lexington 1971).

Krause, C.: Women, ethnicity, and mental health (Institute on Pluralism and Group Identity of the American Jewish Community, New York 1978).

LeGoff, J.: Time, work, and culture in the Middle Ages (University of Chicago Press, Chicago 1980).

LeVine, R.: Culture, behavior, and personality (Aldine Publishing, Chicago 1973).

LeVine, R.; Campbell, D.: The problem of ethnic boundaries; in LeVine, Campbell, Ethnocentrism: theories of conflict, ethnic attitudes, and group behavior (Wiley, New York 1972).

Lieberson, S.: Ethnic patterns in American cities (Free Press/Macmillan, New York 1963).

Litwak, E.: Extended kin relations in an industrial democratic society; in Shanas, Streib, Social structure and the family: generational relations (Prentice-Hall, Englewood Cliffs 1965).

Lopata, H.: Polish-Americans: status competition in an ethnic community (Prentice-Hall, Englewood Cliffs 1976).

Lowenthal, M.F.: Social isolation and mental illness in old age. Am. sociol. Rev. *29:* 54–70 (1964).

Lowenthal, M.F.; Robinson, B.: Social networks and isolation; in Binstock, Shanas, Handbook of aging and the social sciences (Van Nostrand Reinhold, New York 1976).

Lozier, J.; Althouse, R.: Social enforcement of behavior toward elders in an Appalachian mountain settlement. Gerontologist *14:* 67–80 (1974).

Lozier, J.; Althouse, R.: Retirement to the porch in rural Appalachia. Int. J. Aging hum. Dev. *6:* 7–15 (1975).

McDonald, J.: Italy's rural social structure and immigration. Occidente *12:* 437–455 (1956).

McDonald, J.; McDonald, L.: Chain migration, ethnic neighborhood formation, and social networks. Milbank Memorial Fund Q. *42:* 82–97 (1964).

Marshall, V.: Age and awareness of finitude in developmental gerontology. Omega *6:* 113–129 (1975).

Marshall, V.: Last chapters: a sociology of death and dying (Wadsworth Publishing, Belmont 1981).

Mindel, C.; Habenstein, R.: Ethnic families in America (Elsevier, New York 1976).

Mostwin, D.: Emotional needs of elderly Americans of Central and Eastern European background; in Gelfand, Kutznik, Ethnicity aging: theory, research, and policy (Springer, New York 1979).

Munnichs, J.: Old age and finitude: a contribution to psychogerontology (Karger, New York 1966).

Murphy, H.B.M.: Migration and the major mental diseases; in Kantor, Mobility and mental health (Thomas, Springfield 1965).

Murphy, H.B.M.: European cultural offshoots in the New World: differences in their mental hospitalization patterns. I. British, French, and Italian influences. Social Psychiat. *13:* 1–9 (1978).

Neugarten, B.: Personality change in late life: a developmental perspective; in Eisdorfer, Lawton, The psychology of adult development and aging (American Psychological Association, Washington 1973).

Neugarten, B.: Personality and aging; in Birren, Schaie, Handbook of the psychology of aging (Van Nostrand Reinhold, New York 1977).

Neugarten, B.: Time, age, and the life cycle. Am. J. Psychiat. *136:* 887–894 (1979).

Neugarten, B.; Moore, J.W.: The changing age status system; in Neugarten, Middle age and aging (University of Chicago Press, Chicago 1968).

Neugarten, B.; Weinstein, K.: The changing American grandparent. J. Marr. Fam. *26:* 199–204 (1964).

Office of Research and Development: Third annual progress report phase III TRIP evaluation, vol. 2 (West Virginia University, Morgantown 1977).

Odegaard, Q.: Immigration and insanity: a study of mental disease among the Norwegian-born population of Minnesota. Acta psychiat. neurol. scand. *4:* suppl. (1932).

Olson, J.S.: The ethnic dimension in American history (St. Martin's Press, New York 1979).

Opler, M.: Cultural differences in mental disorders: an Italian and Irish contrast in schizophrenias; in Opler, Culture and mental health (Macmillan, New York 1959).

Opler, M.; Singer, J.: Ethnic differences in behavior and psychopathology: Italian and Irish. Int. J. soc. Sci. *2:* 11–22 (1956).

Palmore, E.: When can age, period and cohort be separated? Social Forces *57:* 282–295 (1978).

Palmore, E.: International handbook on aging: contemporary developments and research (Greenwood Press, Westport 1980).

Petersen, W.: Concepts of ethnicity; in Thernstrom, Harvard encyclopedia of American ethnic groups (Harvard University Press, Cambridge 1980).

Plath, D.: Contours of consociation: adult development as discourse; in Baltes, Brim, Life-span development and behavior, vol. III (Academic Press, New York 1980).

Pruchno, R.; Blow, F.; Smyer, M.: Life events and interdependent lives. Hum. Dev. *27:* 31–41 (1984).

Rodeheaver, D.: Going my way: the social environment of elderly travelers (West Virginia University, Morgantown 1981).

Rosow, I.: Social integration of the aged (Free Press, New York 1967).

Rosow, I.: Socialization to old age (University of California Press, Berkeley 1976).

Rubin, E.: The demography of immigration to the United States. Ann. Am. Acad. polit. soc. Sci. *367:* 15–22 (1966).

Sandberg, N.: Ethnic identity and assimilation: the Polish-American community (Praeger Publications, New York 1974).

Schmerhorn, R.: Comparative ethnic relations: a framework for theory and research (Random House, New York 1970).

Schooler, C.: Serfdom's legacy: an ethnic continuum. Am. J. Sociol. *81:* 1265–1286 (1976).

Smith, M.G.: Social and cultural pluralism Ann. N.Y. Acad. Sci. Art. 5, p. 83 (1960).

Spiegel, J.: Transactions: the interplay between individual, family and society (Science House/Aronson, New York 1971).

Stack, C.: All our kin: strategies for survival in a Black community (Harper & Row, New York 1974).

Stein, R.F.: Disturbed youth and ethnic family patterns (State University of New York Press, Albany 1971).

Streib, G.: Old age in Ireland: demographic and sociological aspects; in Cowgill, Holmes, Aging and modernization (Appleton-Century-Crofts, New York 1972).

Sussman, M.B.: The family life of old people; in Binstock, Shanas, Handbook of aging and the social sciences (Van Nostrand Reinhold, New York 1976).

Suttles, G.: Social order of the slums: ethnicity and territory in the city (University of Chicago Press, Chicago 1968).

Thernstrom, S.: Harvard encyclopedia of American ethnic groups (Harvard University Press, Cambridge 1980).

Thomas, W.I.; Znaniecki, F.: The Polish peasant in Europe and America (Knopf, New York 1918–1920).

Treas, J.; Bengtson, V.L.: The demography of mid- and late-life transitions. Ann. Am. Ass. polit. soc. Sci. *464:* 11–21 (1982).

Troll, L.E.: Grandparenting; in Poon, Aging in the 1980s: psychological issues (American Psychological Association, Washington 1980).

Troll, L.E.: Intersections of grandparenting with other life processes. Presented at National Conference on Grandparenthood, Wingspread, Wisc. 1983.

Troll, L.E.; Bengtson, V.L.: Generations in the family; in Burr, Hill, Nye, Reiss, Contemporary theories about the family: research-based theories, vol. 1 (Free Press, New York 1979).

Troll, L.E.; Bengtson, V.L.: Intergenerational relations throughout the life cycle; in Wolman, Handbook of developmental psychology (Prentice-Hall, Englewood Cliffs, 1982).

Troll, L.E.; Miller, S.J.; Atchley, R.C.: Families in later life (Wadsworth, Belmont 1979).

Uhlenhuth, E.; Paykel, E.: Symptom intensity and life events. Archs gen. Psychiat. *25:* 340–347 (1971).

US Bureau of the Census: Characteristics of the population by ethnic origin, Nov. 1969 (US Government Printing Office, Washington 1971).

US Bureau of the Census: Characteristics of the population by ethnic origin, March 1972 and 1971 (US Government Printing Office, Washington 1973).

US Bureau of the Census: Ancestry and language in the United States, Nov. 1979 (US Government Printing Office, Washington 1982).

Van Den Berghe, P.: Race and racism: a comparative perspective (Wiley, New York 1967).

Vecoli, R.: European-Americans: from immigrants to ethnics. Int. Migrat. Rev. *6:* 403–434 (1972).

Verbaro, R.: Philadelphia's south Italians in the 1920s; in Davis, Haller, The peoples of Philadelphia (Temple University Press, Philadelphia 1973).

Wallace, A.F.C.: Revitalization movements. Am. Antrop. *58:* 264–281 (1956).

Ward, D.: Cities and immigrants: a geography of change in nineteenth century America (Oxford University Press, New York 1971).

Waterman, A.: Individualism and interdependence. Am. Psychol. *36:* 762–773 (1981).

Weber, M.: The Protestant ethic and the spirit of capitalism (Scribner, New York 1958/1905).

Weber, M.: Ethnic groups; in Roth, Wittick, Economy and society (Bedminster Press, New York 1968).

Wirth, L.: The ghetto (University of Chicago Press, Chicago 1928).

Wirth, L.: The problem of minority groups; in Linton, The science of man in the world of crisis (Columbia University Press, New York 1945).

Wiseman, R.F.: Spatial aspects of aging (Association of American Geographers, Washington 1978).

Woehrer, C.: The influence of ethnic families on intergenerational relationships and later life transitions. Ann. Am. Acad. polit. soc. Sci. *464:* 65–78 (1982).

Wood, V.: Grandparenthood: an ambiguous role; in Troll, Elders and their families. Generations (Western Gerontological Society, San Francisco 1982).

Wood, V.; Robertson, J.F.: The significance of grandparenthood; in Gubrium, Time, roles, and self in old age (Human Sciences Press, New York 1976).

Wrobel, P.: Our way: family, parish, and neighborhood in a Polish-American community (University of Notre Dame Press, South Bend 1979).

Yancey, W.; Ericksen, E.; Juliani, R.: Emergent ethnicity: a review and formulation. Am. sociol. Rev. *41:* 391–403 (1976).

Zborowski, M.: People in pain (Jossey-Bass, San Francisco 1969).

Ziegler, S.: The family unit and international migration: the perceptions of Italian immigrant children. Int. Migrat. Rev. *11:* 326–333 (1977).

Author Index

Subject Index